HERBAL
REMEDIES

FOR

HEALING

JILL NICE

HERBAL REMEDIES FOR HEALING

A COMPLETE A-Z OF AILMENTS & TREATMENTS

PIATKUS

For Ben and Lotte

The information contained in this book is in no way intended to replace professional medical advice and treatment. If you are in any doubt about your health or you are pregnant, always consult a doctor.

All the treatments suggested in this book will not normally produce adverse side effects. However as there are always exceptions to the rule, the treatments are taken at the reader's sole discretion.

Copyright © 1990 Jill Nice

First published in 1990 by
Judy Piatkus (Publishers) Ltd
5 Windmill St, London W1P 1HF

This edition 1998

The moral right of the author has been asserted

*A catalogue record for this book is available
from the British Library*

ISBN 0–7499–1840–3

Phototypeset in 10/12pt Linotron Baskerville by
Wyvern Typesetting Ltd, Bristol
Printed and bound in Great Britain by
Biddles Ltd, Guildford and King's Lynn

CONTENTS

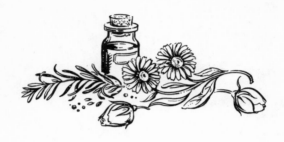

INTRODUCTION

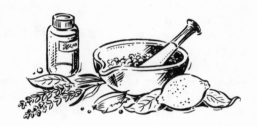

This is a book to be enjoyed and cherished, but above all to be used, and not just in times of illness. More and more people are becoming alarmed at the reliance being made on modern medicines and are seeking natural alternatives, particularly for the most commonplace ailments.

In our great-grandparents' day, when medical advice came dear, if at all, they learned through inherited wisdom how to avoid, ease and cure the myriad of minor ailments which afflicted a household throughout the year. Far from witchcraft with which it was often affiliated, old-fashioned folk wisdom was founded on a combination of local knowledge, psychology, a deep understanding of the values of different herbs and plants and a human desire to cure and relieve suffering.

This book is not intended as a pharmacopoeia for the amateur herbalist or homoeopath but as a gentle and informative handbook for all the family. It is a collection of tried-and-tested old

wives' tales based on herbs and plants. Those which still have relevance today I have updated, and those of dubious benefit I mention for your amusement and amazement only and because they give a curious insight into life in days gone by. I have also included valuable old-fashioned advice on how to avoid many of the more commonplace minor problems and complaints to help ensure the constant good health of your family. In the case of many minor ailments the prevention or cure will often involve a large dose of commonsense.

All the remedies in this book are completely safe and free from the side effects often associated with commercial products. In cases of serious illness they will act as a soothing back up to professional medical care, whilst for minor ailments they will provide pleasant, effective alternatives to commercially produced products.

All the remedies are easy to prepare using readily available ingredients. What's more, the psychological advan-

1

tage for both patient and nurse of a made-to-measure home-made (and even homegrown) remedy or comforter will outweigh the slight inconvenience of having to prepare it.

I am neither a medic nor a homoeopath and I would be the first person to seek professional medical advice when my family or I are ill. Consequently this book is not intended to replace your family doctor whose advice should still be sought whenever that unwelcome visitor – illness – enters your door. It can, however, be comfortably used alongside professional medical care.

A Note to the Reader

Although making one's own remedies and recipes is a fascinating and rewarding business it is worth remembering that in order to obtain the best results and to be able to keep them for as long as is possible a few simple rules should be adhered to.

Herbs

Herbs that are gathered fresh, particularly those from the wild, must be picked from areas that are free from contamination caused by exhaust fumes, dogs, pesticides etc. It makes sense, therefore, to grow a few herbs – in pots if necessary – in your garden.

Always try to pick before the herb has flowered and in the early morning before the sun is at its highest and the volatile oils are destroyed.

If your only source of seed, leaf and root is from a herbalist then make sure that they are from a reliable source. Some actually specify that they have been grown without the aid of artificial fertilizers or pesticides.

Be sure to buy only those that are recommended for consumption as opposed to those intended for pot pourri.

Always use fresh ingredients and not those which have been lurking in a dank cupboard for several months.

Dried herbs are more concentrated than fresh and therefore, as a general rule, quantities should be halved.

Herbal Teas

When preparing herbal teas, unless otherwise stated make in the proportions of 15g(½oz) dried or 25g(1oz) fresh herb to 600ml(1 pint) boiling water.

Containers and Storage

All containers should be immaculately clean, dry and sterile. Wash out with very hot water and either dry with a clean cloth or, in the case of glass jars and bottles, leave to dry upside down in a cool oven. If you have to use metal lids then make sure that they are plastic lined otherwise you run the risk of the carefully prepared contents reacting with the metal and causing unappetising and potentially dangerous results.

It is advisable to make up all your lotions and potions in fairly small quantities. Unless otherwise stated keep all your home-made products in a cool dark place. Once opened they should be kept in the refrigerator. Keep all creams and salves in the refrigerator in hot weather.

Essential Oils

These are extremely potent and should not normally be used undiluted. Always follow the instructions given for diluting them in a base oil (such as sunflower oil) or dispersing them in water.

Not all brands of essential oils are intended for internal use, so check before you buy.

ACHES AND PAINS IN THE BODY

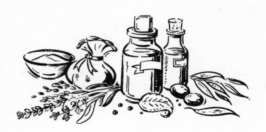

CRAMP

Despite the agonizing pain of a cramped limb it is only a muscular spasm caused by either unaccustomed exercise, strenuous movement or paradoxically a prolonged period spent in one position which may have impaired the circulation of blood to the muscle. The muscle, usually in the calf, becomes knotted and when any attempt is made to move it becomes doubly rigid and painful. Vigorous rubbing and massage soon dispel the tension but if the limb still feels stiff and aches then this should be followed by hot compresses until the muscle moves quite freely.

For those people in the past who suffered from cramp there were many sovereign remedies to guarantee immunity: a cork placed beneath the pillow or a core of brimstone in the pocket; a sheep's kneecap, a snake or eelskin band tied above the knee, or the supple strands of sorcerer's violet (periwinkle) twined about the afflicted limb. All these were recommended to charm away the devils that made you 'gate-legged'. Swapping one's shoes for some other poor soul's might seem a particularly unphilanthropic instance of pain transference but suffering from night cramps has a debilitating effect which warps the soul. A stone bottle at the bottom of the bed to flex the feet against during the night seems a sensible idea but less so the practice of placing a potato between the mattress and limb, which could surely do no more than ensure a restless night and thus an active circulation.

Persistent night cramps are often caused by poor circulation and are a double menace because they disturb a good night's sleep, so give a thought to the old-fashioned solution still in use today of strapping a small magnet to the most susceptible limb before retiring at night. However, if night cramp is the rule rather than the exception it is advisable to seek professional advice. Stomach cramps are frequently caused

3

by eating in an unnatural position or whilst in a state of tension and can be particularly painful and frightening if the victim is convinced that something worse is wrong.

The pain of cramp should not be underestimated. Some period pain suffered by women is no more than a form of cramp yet it will send the afflicted to bed with a hot-water bottle and a glass of hot gin and peppermint cordial until the pain subsides, whilst children are appalled at the ferocity of a 'stitch' which is cramp in the side caused by excessive running and for which the only cure is to drop to one knee and touch the other raised knee with the forehead whilst reciting the alphabet.

Generally speaking, cramp is an instant but temporary protest from the body at being overexerted. However, if it persists it may indicate a dietary deficiency. Vitamins including C, D, E and B_{12} and the minerals calcium, magnesium and salt are all very necessary to ensure a smooth-moving body. Athletes frequently suffer from cramp caused by a salt deficiency created by excess sweating.

Relaxing Rubs and Poultices

● *Tincture of myrrh* If rubbed directly into the muscle or sprinkled on to a hot, damp cloth and laid on the limb will bring quick relief.

● *Essential oil of cloves* Seven drops of this spicy aromatic oil added to 1 teaspoon of sunflower oil and massaged into the length of the muscle is warming and comforting.

● *Essential oil of camomile* A few drops diluted in 1 tablespoon of sunflower oil and rubbed into the painful area of neck and upper shoulder has a relaxing effect.

● *Pennyroyal* Either a few drops of the oil in 1 tablespoon of sunflower oil, or

the crushed leaves of this old-fashioned mint, rubbed into an aching limb is a time-honoured Fenland remedy.

● *Athlete's massage oil* Two drops each of the essential oils of lemon, pine and juniper shaken with 1 tablespoon of sunflower oil may be used as a massage oil prior to exercise.

● *A green poultice* The white part of a leek chopped, pounded and warmed in white vinegar then placed on a hot cloth and applied to the area of the lower rib was by some considered to be the definitive answer to a persistent 'stitch', but then others might have advocated the use of cabbage leaves strapped to the side. Both cabbages and leeks figure very strongly in the folk medicine of those damp regions where the inhabitants might have suffered most severely from muscular complaints. I do, however, believe that as both vegetables are valuable sources of vitamins and minerals the sufferers would have been wiser to have eaten them.

Soothing Baths

● *Oil of thyme, rosemary or horse chestnut* (an essential ingredient of *Badedas*) Any of these oils when added a few drops at a time to a pleasantly hot bath will help prevent night cramps.

● *Warm sitz bath* A bath in which you sit, with knees raised, immersed in warm water (which may be plain or herbal) up to the navel and swathed in towels for 10 to 20 minutes is a recommended cure for stomach and menstrual cramps.

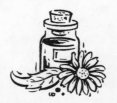

Drink and Diet

A warm milky drink before going to bed will help .to ensure a quiet night free from cramp. Try the following posset which contains a combination of nourishing ingredients.

Posset
2 tablespoons clear honey
1 glass warm buttermilk
juice of 1 lemon

Dissolve the honey in the buttermilk then beat in the lemon juice. Drink slowly but immediately.

● *Blackstrap molasses or honey* Stir either of these up in a glass of hot water to give instant comfort to children. In the long-term both are valuable additions to the diet.
● *Nettle tea* Nettles contain a high proportion of mineral salts and vitamins which can alleviate cramp if taken regularly. Take 50g(2oz) of dried nettle leaves and boil for three minutes in 1 litre(1¾ pints) of water. Leave to infuse for 10 minutes and drink one cup three times a day.
● *Mineral salts* Sufferers from cramp appear to be deficient in mineral salts and a regular intake of foods high in those necessary salts is to be recommended especially in the case of children and people past middle age. The following greenstuffs were all an integral part of ancient recipes and remedies for cramp. They are also

mildly diuretic but, much more to the point, they make a delicious salad.

Green Salad
crisp green lettuce
watercress
shredded spinach
shredded nasturtium leaves
shredded dandelion leaves
chopped fennel leaves and bulb
salad dressing

Juggle the proportions of each ingredient to suit individual tastes. Pound some garlic, honey and mint together to make the dressing and garnish with a nasturtium flower (nasturtium is a natural antibiotic).

● *Rhubarb* Another ancient cure-all recommended to prevent cramp. The juice, sweetened with honey and diluted with sparkling mineral water, is a really delicious drink which acts as a deterrent rather than a cure.

HOUSEMAID'S KNEE

Bursitis, the painful swelling of the knee joint, should not be ascribed to housemaids alone. It is a condition associated with the use and abuse of the knees and is indeed also known as clergyman's or parson's knee. There were, as might be expected, a myriad of domestic remedies for what was and still is a most debilitating and painful complaint, ranging from the doubtful applications of hot clay, warm wax, onions or seaweed to the even more curious practice of flagellating the knee with nettles whilst reciting a rune – after which exorcism the original pain must have appeared as naught.

Nevertheless, there was a fundamental element of wisdom in these strange remedies. Hot clay, wax and hot and cold compresses are still in common use today for these kinds of injuries, particularly amongst sportsmen, and health hydros and spas make a special feature of their use. Onions were prescribed for a great many illnesses, mainly because of their antiseptic properties, but in this particular instance would have been better employed in the stomach where the mineral and vitamin content might have acted, in the long-term, as a preventative against bursitis. Another favourite poultice for painful joints was a liberal plastering of seaweed. Presumably the iodine which seaweed contains was thought to be of benefit. At one time a large amount of iodine itself would have been pasted upon the knee in the belief that the resulting blisters released internal poisons!

Rather than scouring the knee with birch twigs or nettles take a bath in the leaves of either or substitute eucalyptus. If you cannot obtain the large quantity of leaves required use instead a spot or two of eucalyptus oil in the bath, drink birch leaf tonic and make a comforting and nourishing nettle soup. These are all very pleasant remedies which require far less masochistic zeal.

Once the knees become susceptible to injury bursitis will recur, so take avoiding action and do as the professionals do: carpet layers wear thick pads around their knees; gardeners kneel on well-wadded mats (old hot-water bottles, snug in velvet jackets, make excellent kneelers). Whether the condition exists or not, prevention is always better than cure.

There is a condition which is similar

to bursitis but which affects the elbow. It is limited to certain groups of people where it is known as toper's or bar fly's elbow!

Soothing Lotions and Poultices

It is not advisable to massage swollen or inflamed joints too vigorously although gentle movement is recommended. Bring initial relief from pain by bathing with cold compresses followed by a warm poultice or apply alternate hot and cold compresses.

● *Witch hazel* This old-fashioned lotion applied on a damp cloth will cool the joint. Air travellers might like to note that commercial face-freshening tissues which can be bought in tins and which are soaked with a mild astringent will bring exquisite relief to hot knees aching from too many cramped flying hours.

● *Comfrey poultice* The soaked leaves when applied as a warm poultice will relieve the pain of any swollen joint.

● *Wintergreen oil* A few drops of this pungent oil mixed with 1 teaspoon of sunflower oil, rubbed gently over the afflicted area then covered with a thick bandage, will do much to soothe the pain.

● *Housemaid's liniment* One coffee spoon each of the essential oils of lavender, marjoram, eucalyptus and rosemary mixed with 5 teaspoons of sunflower oil can be used to very gently massage the knee several times a day.

Drink and Diet

Bursitis is usually caused by overuse of the poor old knees or elbow but it is also a condition which can be accelerated by or as a result of a poor diet. Avoid carbohydrates and eat plenty of fresh fruit and vegetables, strong green leaves, oranges, beans, peas, kelp, fish, wheatgerm, apricots, molasses, prunes, brewer's yeast and lots of fresh, clear water. Reduce or try to avoid altogether tea, coffee, alcohol and cigarettes. Remember that it is doubly important to watch what you eat during any period of enforced inactivity.

• *Lovage tea* A handful of this delicious and savoury herb brewed in 300ml(½ pint) of good chicken stock or water has a diuretic effect which will help to dispel toxic wastes from the body.

• *Sarsaparilla* This North American tonic drink beloved of cowboy heroes is, if taken regularly, a good preventative against pain and swelling in the joints.

• *Sage leaves* Eaten every day these were believed by country women to keep the joints supple and the body youthful. Chop them up with a low-fat soft cheese and spread on wholemeal bread.

TENNIS ELBOW

Tendonitis is an inflammation of the muscles and tendons, strained and jarred by strenuous sport, hence the names tennis elbow and golfer's elbow. It is not, however, a modern complaint but one endured for centuries by men and women who undertook heavy manual work such as lifting, washing utensils and cooking pots, wringing clothes, scrubbing floors or taking part in the labours of harvesting. In the mines workers suffered from inflamed elbows caused by resting the weight of the body upon their points, hence miner's elbow which was in fact a condition more akin to bursitis. Children who lean upon the points of their elbows whilst concentrating on schoolwork may also suffer the same painful inflammation of the bursa.

Tennis elbow may take a long time to clear up but the pain can be relieved by the constant application of cold compresses or in severe cases by hot and cold compresses applied alternately. Warm poultices, particularly of comfrey leaves, can also be applied to ease the inflammation and swelling and once this has subsided oil of comfrey may be rubbed very gently into the area. Although opinions differ it is generally considered best to keep the affected arm immobilized in a sling.

SPRAINS

As a result of a twist in the opposite direction to that in which the rest of their body was travelling most people at some time in their lives sprain some part of their anatomy. Painful though it may be the injury is on most occasions temporary and relief is rapidly achieved by the application of cold compresses and where possible a supporting bandage and rest.

The old favourite of wrapping layers of brown paper, well pasted with vinegar, around a badly sprained ankle ensured a rock-hard cast and almost total immobility – a novel idea for overactive children which would not only render them *hors de combat* but also impose upon them a hero's status. Children in pursuit of each other, playing leapfrog, catching a ball or turning cartwheels do manage to sprain the most amazing parts of their bodies. Cold compresses of sweet-smelling witch hazel followed by a gentle rub with rosemary oil (see page 21) and applied sympathetic attention will usually cure the matter in minutes. On the beach a twisted ankle can be temporarily eased by a bandage of bladderwrack (seaweed). By the time the novelty has worn off the pain has usually disappeared as well. Gardeners might like to consider the countryman's remedy of fresh green cabbage leaves, rid of their thick central vein, softened and heated by blanching in boiling water, wrapped around the sprained limb.

Soothing Lotions and Oils

- *Tincture of arnica* Up to 10 drops of arnica in a cup of cold water and applied on a compress reduces swelling and brings out bruising. Do not use undiluted or on broken skin.
- *Comfrey lotion* Steep the injured limb in a bowl of strong comfrey tea to ease the pain.
- *Epsom salts* A bowl or bath of pleasantly warm water into which has been stirred a good handful of Epsom salts is a time-honoured remedy for sprains. To make it even more pleasant and effective add either a good handful of thyme or pennyroyal or a few drops of the essential oil.
- *Rosemary, lavender, sage, thyme or marigold* Up to 8 drops of any one of these healing essential oils added to 1 tablespoon of sunflower oil and massaged into the painful area will, over a period of days, bring relief without soreness.
- *Garlic* Pounded in olive oil, rubbed into the sprain and then covered with a warm bandage, this is an effective if malodorous healer.
- *Turpentine and sunflower* Two tablespoons of sunflower oil shaken in a jar with 1 tablespoon of oil of turpentine is an old-fashioned liniment for sprains given to me by a vet, but I can assure you that it works very well on human beings too.
- *Camphor rub* Mix in the proportions of 1 teaspoon of oil of camphor to 1 cupful of sunflower oil. Camphor is

believed to have strange powers which will send pendulums and dials haywire so be careful upon whose wrists it is rubbed.
- *Poacher's liniment* Mix together 1 teaspoon each of wintergreen (natural wintergreen is prohibitively expensive so use the synthetic form), camphor, clove and turpentine oils with 1 cup of sunflower oil. Whilst this excellent rub may have healed sprains caused by fleeing the gamekeeper in the dark of night I cannot help but feel that that same gamekeeper along with all the poacher's intended victims would have smelt him coming from a long way off.

Poultices

- *Vervain or parsley* Either herb, macerated in hot water and placed as a warm poultice, will soothe sprains and stitches.
- *Hot soured milk* Apply it as a poultice on a warm cloth.
- *Onion and honey* Onion, finely chopped and mixed with honey, was used to heal a multitude of hurts.
- *Harvester's remedy* A rag soaked in cider and wrapped around the sprained limb was an easy and effective bandage for countrymen at work. Cider vinegar is equally effective.

GANGLIA

A ganglion is an odd swelling which rises up under the skin on the wrist, the back of the hand or the top of the foot. There seems to be no rhyme or reason for its occurring and although ganglia are quite small and painless professional advice should always be sought when mysterious lumps and bumps appear. The old-fashioned method of dispersing a ganglion was to thump it mightily with the family Bible. This is not to be recommended.

ARTHRITIS

Arthritis, in the most simplistic terms, affects the joints and bones. Some specialists believe that living in a damp, cold climate increases the likelihood of becoming afflicted with this very painful and debilitating condition; others ascribe it to overuse, for example typists whose fingers become knotted, athletes with swollen knees and troublesome hips, ballerinas with painful feet. Occasionally it can be caused by a bad fall, a severe jolt or the trauma of an accident. One of the interesting aspects of arthritis is the higher proportion of women to men who suffer from it and it is reasonable to believe that this is as a result of the hormonal changes which take place during the menopause, causing not only a physical decline but leading also to emotional upheavals which in turn may lead to a state of unhappy introspection.

It was at one time believed that poisons in the system were created by bitterness, intolerance and the brooding desire for revenge and that as this type of unhealthy anger could not thrive in an atmosphere of love and forgiveness the antidote should be religious ritual in the form of confirmation, as many times as was necessary, to rid the body of its evil arthritis-forming toxins! I cannot help but feel that this was a bit hard on the poor old vicar who must surely have despaired at finding that his sermons upon 'loving thy neighbour' were persistently falling on deaf ears. Nevertheless it is true to say that emotional stress and anxiety do leave their physical mark upon the body and perhaps we should not scoff at those chauvinistic old psychologists of yesteryear.

Anodynes and Sovereign Cures

- *Devil's claw* (*Harpagophytum procumbens*) This strange thorny plant from Africa gains its name from its vicious habit of impaling unwary travellers. It is believed to cure arthritis and it can be bought in both tablet and tea-bag form. It is wise before embarking upon any course of treatment to take careful note of the instructions or to consult a homoeopathic practitioner.
- *Aspirin* This still seems to be the only true, tried and tested anodyne for arthritis.
- *Oil of evening primrose* It is now believed that if women start taking evening primrose oil during and after the menopause they will never suffer from arthritis. It is also thought to be able to arrest an existing condition.
- *Cider vinegar and honey* One teaspoon of each in hot water taken first thing in the morning will reduce the chances of arthritis.
- *Honey and lemon* Some fruits should not be eaten by arthritis sufferers but lemon juice has a beneficial effect. Take daily the juice of 1 lemon in hot water sweetened with honey.
- *Agrimony tea or willow bark tea* An infusion of either taken daily and persevered with over a long period of time will bring relief. Agrimony and willow both contain a fair amount of salicylic acid which is the vital component of aspirin.
- *Nettle and sage tea or catnip tea* Both

are excellent and pleasant-tasting teas which have a mildly sedative and regenerative effect, relieving tension and improving the state of mind. For other teas which will allay anxiety and thus improve a painful arthritic condition see **Anxiety**.

- *Swimming* One of the best ways of ensuring a lithe and healthy body is to swim daily. Taking a bathe daily or as often as is possible will relieve arthritis. Spa treatments, where one can swim and is fasted on natural spring water are considered by many to be far better than any other treatments and can be repeated regularly if circumstances allow, without adverse side effects. Indoor heated swimming pools and a self-inflicted fast, drinking only a good quality bottled mineral water, may not be so luxurious but will bring the same benefits.

Oils, Liniments and Poultices

- *Compresses* Try a red flannel wrapped gently around a painful joint or alternate hot and cold compresses left on overnight as soon as the twinges start.
- *Olive oil* A gentle massage with warm olive oil as soon as the pain starts is cheap and effective.
- *Garlic, juniper, lavender, cajuput, sage, rosemary, thyme, or sassafras* Any one of these oils diluted in the proportions of one part to 10 parts of olive oil and used to massage the painful joint will bring immense relief.

Liniment for Arthritis
2 drops essential oil of cloves
3 drops essential oil of eucalyptus
3 drops oil of wintergreen (synthetic)
7 drops oil of camphor B.P.
2 tablespoons olive oil

Shake together thoroughly and use to massage the afflicted joint.

Diet

There are many conflicting theories which arise over how much the diet creates or affects arthritis. Nevertheless it would be safe to say that when the condition becomes more painful an examination of the diet may reveal certain adverse factors. Red meat and dairy produce are destructive whilst a vegetarian diet, or one including fish, with plenty of raw fruit and vegetables can do nothing but good. There are those who swear that stewed fruit creates havoc whilst others believe that chocolate or refined carbohydrate have an equally devastating effect. An extra supplement of calcium, zinc and vitamin C is often recommended and worth trying at an early stage. See also **Rheumatism**, **Constipation** and **Catarrhal Infections** for more information on food and drink.

- *Cabbage juice* This surprisingly pleasant drink is also frequently suggested to alleviate catarrh so that one cannot help but wonder if the two conditions are connected.
- *Garlic* Stringing garlic bulbs about the afflicted limb was a strong device offered by the wise women. Several garlic cloves chewed daily are an excellent idea but if this is too ghastly to contemplate try garlic perles or capsules.
- *Celery* All parts eaten raw are considered to be effective. Celery contains a fair quantity of minerals and it is also a valuable diuretic.
- *Potatoes* There is an ancient recipe, one of many which come from the Fenland region of Britain where they undoubtedly suffered from a high per-

centage of damp-induced ailments, which suggests drinking the juice of raw potatoes seasoned mightily with crushed mustard seed! I view eating raw potatoes with severe misgivings and would suggest instead that potatoes baked in their jackets and filled with cottage cheese, tinned tuna, parsley and dill will do you far more good.

● *Nettles* Nettle tea is an excellent idea and so is the following recipe.

Nettle Soup

3 tablespoons finely chopped onion
2 cloves garlic, finely chopped
4 tablespoons sunflower oil
1 tablespoon flour
600ml(1 pint) chicken stock or water
450g(1lb) fresh young nettle tops
600ml(1 pint) skimmed milk
salt and freshly ground black pepper
chopped parsley and chives to garnish

Place the onions and garlic in a large pan with the oil and cook gently until they are transparent but not brown. Stir in the flour followed by the stock or water, a little at a time, until you have a thick, well-blended sauce. Add the carefully washed nettle tops, cover and simmer until they are soft. Purée in a blender. Return the soup to the pan and reheat, making sure that you do not bring it to the boil again and adding as much milk as is necessary for the thickness you prefer. Season to taste and garnish.

RHEUMATISM

The word rheumatism relates to a disease of a moist nature leading to watery deposits in the joints. When most people lived and laboured in the country the varied aches and pains put under the heading of rheumatism were caused by physically stressful work, carried out in adverse weather conditions and aggravated by damp, ill-heated houses. There were a score of ancient remedies to alleviate or prevent this occurring, many of which are in common use today. The most noteworthy example is that of wearing a copper bangle, a worldwide custom much derided by men of science who would find it even more difficult to explain why a potato carried in the pocket becomes increasingly fossilized as the rheumatic condition improves. Scoff one might, but commonsense was paramount when a loss of livelihood was at stake.

Washed wool beneath the feet would keep the damp from creeping through the soles of the shoes although sulphur powder in the foot of the stocking owed more, I suspect, to its hellishly hot associations than its mild antiseptic properties. Beating the body with holly is less comprehensible than beating with nettles or rolling naked in a nettle bed as nettles contain formic acid which is considered helpful in the treatment of rheumatism. It is for the same reason that the stings of angry bees were considered beneficial. Better, perhaps, a bee sting than coming to terms with swallowing live spiders or carrying a collection of moles' feet around in the breast pocket, for neither of which I can find an explanation. There may be more to be said for the practice of stuffing eelskins with lavender and burying them in layers of peat and mint, after which, suitably macerated, they were tied above the right knee of a man or the left knee of a woman. A fatty eelskin full of warming, antiseptic lavender, impregnated with oils and minerals from its earthy incarceration where it must, presumably, have lost some of its smell, would probably have been quite cosy! It would have been more comfortable, at any rate, than a massage of searing mustard oil or a fiery rub of red peppers in oil from the North American Indians.

Warmth, not surprisingly, figured strongly in the treatments for rheumatic pains. Boiled sea water applied on compresses and the floury contents of potatoes baked in their jackets made use of local ingredients both of which contain minerals which might have penetrated into the painful joint, whilst flannel cloth laid on the body and smoothed over with an iron, hot from the fire, had much in common with today's treatment of Turkish baths or saunas followed by a good massage. Hot baths, hot-water bottles and even hair dryers have all been used to comfort aching limbs although the thought of yielding up one's body to electrical treatments with the names of Galvanism and Faradism make one's hair stand on end. The most pleasant remedy that I can bring to mind is to indulge in a warm, soothing bath, rub the aching joint with a therapeutic liniment and retire to a well-heated bed with a good book and a warm drink.

Baths and Poultices

- *Epsom salts* Whether the quantity recommended be in kilos or cups, Epsom salts added to the bath water has always been considered an important method of easing rheumatic pain. One cupful should be enough.
- *Essential oil of rosemary, pine, lavender or juniper* Add a few drops to the bath water, with or without Epsom salts.
- *Seaweed extract or powder* Long believed to be valuable because of its iodine content, it will ensure a healing and invigorating bath.
- *Mustard and cayenne* One dessert-spoon of each whisked into the bath water should have the desired effect.

Oils and Liniments

The most famous remedy for aches and pains is the classic Tiger Balm – that aromatic and effective blend of camphor, cajuput, cassia, cloves, menthol and peppermint. There are, however, a host of proprietary brands of creams and liniments on the market and some very good ones that you can make yourself. The majority of the following remedies are effective on all aches, pains, sprains and arthritis.
- *Essential oil of peppermint or coriander* A few drops of either of these sweet-smelling oils in a tablespoon of almond oil and massaged in is exotic and soothing. Several drops in a glass of hot water will also improve the digestive disorders that many rheumatic people suffer from.
- *Eucalyptus, camphor and wintergreen oils* The following recipe is the most effective liniment of all and works wonders on bruises, sprains, pulled muscles and unbroken chilblains, to name but a few complaints.

A Cream for Aches and Pains
4 teaspoons emulsifying wax
4 teaspoons coconut oil
1 teaspoon each oil of eucalyptus,
camphor and wintergreen (synthetic)
½ teaspoon each oil of clove and
juniper
4 teaspoons almond or sunflower oil
4 tablespoons purified water
2 teaspoons each tinctures of arnica,
myrrh and benzoin
2 tablespoons witch hazel

Warm the wax and oils together in one bain-marie and the water, tinctures and witch hazel together in another. When the wax and oils are melted remove both bowls from the heat. Beat the liquid slowly into the oils and continue stirring briskly until nearly cold. Pour into clean, dry jars. Seal when cold.

Camphor Rub
¼ teaspoon each camphor and mustard powder
300ml(½ pint) pure oil of turpentine
300ml(½ pint) sunflower oil
300ml(½ pint) rubbing alcohol

Dissolve the camphor and mustard powder in the turpentine. Pour into a large glass jar and add the oil and alcohol. Shake well together and use to massage aching limbs and wheezy chests. The area anointed must be kept well covered and warm.

Diet

Rheumatic conditions are often exacerbated by constipation and kidney disorders. Therefore it is important to regulate the diet and in aggravated circumstances to avoid all tea, coffee, alcohol, white sugar and bread, food additives and acid fruit with the exception of lemon which has been proven to be beneficial. It does appear that stewed fruit has a worse effect upon the system than fresh.

These are only basic ideas to ease those pains which appear to the layman as 'rheumaticky' but there are certain conditions which do require specific diets. Eating the right food all the time can help to prevent rheumatism occurring. Plenty of good green vegetables are essential. Kale, nettles (in soup), watercress, parsley, fennel and sorrel are all particularly good as they are high in minerals and vitamins as well as being gently laxative and diuretic.

- *Celery* Make a celery soup or simply stew the celery gently in milk or stock. Some sources advocate chewing celery seed but this can be harmful if done to excess, particularly when pregnant. Celery as a foodstuff has no unpleasant side effects.
- *Onion drink* Chop 3 washed but unpeeled onions into 1 litre (1¾ pints) of water and boil gently in a covered saucepan for 15 minutes. Strain and drink one cup morning or night. This is not quite as bad as it sounds but a little antisocial.
- *Cloves of garlic* Several cloves of garlic pounded in olive oil with parsley and eaten on coarse brown bread is somewhat more appetizing, in fact quite delicious.
- *Kelp* Powdered seaweed, sprinkled on broth or soup, contains many valuable minerals.
- *Apples* An unpeeled apple a day will keep the body in good working order. Grated apple mixed with raw oats and yoghurt is a good way to start the day.
- *Cider* This has to be good, rough cider, not the commercial varieties from which all natural goodness has been eradicated. One to 2 glasses of cider daily or 1 teaspoon of cider vinegar act as both a preventative and cure. Cider is also good for the kidneys.
- *Juniper berries* Three chewed daily are said to prevent rheumatism.

Anodynes

- *Blackcurrant leaf tea* Crumple up a handful of fresh or dried leaves into a teapot of boiling water and infuse for 10 minutes. The dried leaves are stronger than the fresh.
- *Infusion of pansy or marigold flowers* Taken three to four times daily, this brings relief probably because, as in the

case of blackcurrant leaves, these trusted herbs clear the blood of impurities.

- *Dandelion tea* Boil 25g(1oz) of dandelion root for 20 minutes in 900ml(1½ pints) of water then strain and drink half a cup twice daily during the period in which the joints are uncomfortable.
- *Poppy tea* The prescribing of this old-fashioned tea as a pain killer might well lead to a crisis of confidence with the local constabulary!
- *White willow* Aspirin is obtained from white willow in the form of salicin and, as yet, no better modern answer has been found to replace this ancient remedy. It is interesting to note that, as is the case with so many herbal remedies, the cure, willow, grows best in those areas where the ailment flourishes (in this case damp areas).

LUMBAGO

Lumbago is a rheumatic pain in the lumbar region of the back and it is caused primarily by unaccustomed overexertion – moving furniture, digging virgin soil, ill-advised board sailing and so on. Although the remedies and recipes given for rheumatism and arthritis can be used equally effectively to bring relief to lumbago sufferers the traditional cure for lumbago was for a child who was born feet first to stand upon the victim's back. More latterly, however, small Japanese ladies have been found to perform this same service, a treatment which has been variously described as sheer bliss and toe-torture of the highest order. Because of the easy access to that area of the back and the fact that the patient has, by force of circumstances, to lie flat on his or her stomach until the pulled

muscle, muscle spasm or sprained muscle or ligaments right themselves, there are several poultices which can relieve the pain and speed recovery. Otherwise it is just a matter of time.

Poultices and Other Pleasant Painkillers

- *Whole oats* Cook to a mash with vinegar and apply as hot as possible.
- *Vervain* Soak a handful of fresh, crushed vervain in cold water for 10 minutes then boil briefly in a little wine vinegar and apply on a cloth as hot as possible. Vervain tea is supremely tranquillizing and refreshing and can do nothing but good for the beleaguered spirit – both that of patient and of the nurse.
- *Cabbage leaves* Boil in milk until they become a jelly, spread on a cloth and apply hot then leave overnight.
- *Juniper oil* Place 100g(4oz) juniper berries in a glass jar with 500ml(17 fl oz) olive oil. Seal tightly and leave to stand in the sun for one month, shaking daily. Use as a massage oil for all aches and pains, rheumatic or otherwise. After massaging cover with a wad of cotton wool saturated with the oil and bandage in place.
- *Lumbago embrocation* Shake together 1 cup each of vinegar and turpentine with 1 dessertspoon of powdered camphor and 1 whole egg. Keep refrigerated and use quickly.

GOUT

Gout is caused by an excess of uric acid which accumulates in the system forming crystals which are caught in the spaces between the joints and cause inflammation and irritation. Thus an excruciating pain is created in thumb, knee or elbow and, most commonly, the big toe. The area affected becomes painful overnight, swells, turns a deep, throbbing red. This is something that can happen to anyone although it is frequently viewed with hilarity by one's friends who traditionally view it as a form of divine retribution for too much high living and overindulgence.

The best and most devious remedy that I have heard of to date is that of advising the patient to get undressed in the early evening hours, swathe him or herself in blankets and sit in hot water up to the knees prior to retiring to bed before 10 o'clock. Sweating will reduce the uric acid in the body and make the condition more comfortable but more to the point this remedy kept the patient immobilized and at the mercy of the nurse who then removed all alcoholic nightcaps from within reach. The trouble is that the pain is so awful that a stiff drink promises the only anodyne, but alcohol, rich or acid foods and red meat are all absolutely taboo. Working on the principle that 'what kills may cure' the wealthy society of yesteryear wrapped the afflicted toe around with raw red beef, a civilized improvement on the Tibetan remedy of rancid milk, butter and cow dung.

People who suffer from gout are, understandably, extremely bad tempered and undoubtedly resent the sniggers it causes. Sympathy and a visit to a professional practitioner are essential as gout may be just a visible symptom of a more serious underlying ailment. Do not take painkillers, not even aspirin, unless prescribed. Make life as comfortable as possible by keeping the foot raised and wadded with cotton wool to protect it from being knocked. Pleasant soothing herbal teas, a light diet and any entertainment guaranteed to keep the blood pressure down are the best

answers although there are alternatives.

A poultice may seem a practical method of curing gout but the likelihood of a patient welcoming one's approach with a view to applying a hot poultice or hot and cold compresses is, as has been suggested, remote in the extreme. Goutwort (goutweed or ground elder), as the name implies, was considered the ultimate remedy for the aching joints caused by gout, rheumatism and sciatica. A poultice of the leaves will help but a more appropriate solution would be to eat the leaves in salads as a preventative measure although they have a slightly disagreeable flavour unless picked very young. Bran and vinegar poultice or tallow and garlic shared equal popularity with a thick covering of treacle or honey applied on a flannel cloth. However, the most highly prized infusion with which to bathe a gouty toe was made from meadow saffron which, in the language of flowers, means 'my best days are over' – a message hardly conducive to improving the patient's spirits!

Dandelion and burdock tonic, which tastes not unlike beer, is a pleasant enough drink for those whose alcoholic taste buds are suffering withdrawal symptoms but at the same time it acts as a valuable diuretic. Apples, onions, pears, mustard seeds and juniper berries were all considered necessary to the patient's diet whilst sweetcorn, cooked with its tassels on, is still used extensively in some parts of Europe. It is quite clear, however, that any drink or

food which might be suggested as a cure for gout is, in effect, either a mild sedative or a diuretic.

FROZEN SHOULDER

Frozen shoulder or fibrositis is a condition where the shoulder becomes stiff and painful deep within the muscle. The major reasons for its occurring are physical strain (such as pulling a muscle), tension, sitting in a draught, anxiety and emotional stress. A prime example of do-it-yourself fibrositis is driving yourself, with the window of the car open, to an important appointment for which you are already late. The best way of loosening up the shoulder muscles is to stretch the neck, wiggle the shoulders and squeeze the shoulder blades together. Stretching out and forward with the arms and punching the air high above the head also relieves tension. The teas suggested to relieve **Anxiety** will all help, as will the liniments and embrocations listed under **Cramp** and **Rheumatism**.

BACK PROBLEMS

Most back trouble is non-specific, meaning that it has no direct cause. **Lumbago**, **Rheumatism**, **Frozen Shoulder** and **Sciatica** can all be identified but apart from a slipped disc, which is a slipped or prolapsed disc in the backbone, and spondylosis, a stiffening of the backbone particularly in the neck resulting in a loss of easy movement, many back troubles are sporadic and vague. Pregnancy and heavy periods can cause chronic backache, and so can constipation. Rest and warmth in all cases seem to bring the most comfort, or maybe we should fol-

low the example of the old wives and run a hot iron across a sufferer's back or rub it with methylated spirit and dust it with starch – an idea which is still used even today in some gymnasiums. Any of the creams and liniments in this chapter will bring relief.

SCIATICA

Sciatica is caused by pressure on the sciatic nerve where it leaves the spinal cord. It is usually felt in the top centre of the buttock, through which a fiery pain shoots and continues on down the back of the thigh and towards the ankle. Any sudden movement or any attempt to bend increases the pain. Herbals of many years ago graphically described sciatica as 'boneshave' and one way of ridding yourself of it was to take a straight stick and lie in a preordained position by a running stream into which you chanted a rune designed to remove the infirmity from you to your stick. Although sciatic pain is not quite the same as rheumatism and arthritis most of the remedies given in this chapter will soothe and relax this condition very well. There are also one or two fairly specific ones to try.

Poultices and Potions

- *Ivy leaf poultice* Take 2 handfuls of ivy (*Hedera helix*), chop finely and mix with twice its volume of bran. Stir to a paste with 250ml(scant ½ pint) of water and leave in an enamel pan over a low heat for 10 minutes. Apply on a cloth and leave for at least half an hour.

● *Fenugreek seeds* Crushed and mixed to a mash with boiling hot milk these make a very effective poultice for rheumatism and especially for localized pains such as sciatica. The mixture will also soothe bruises and swellings.

● *White clover and lime tea* Mixed together or taken separately both teas are pleasurably relaxing.

● *Black radish or horseradish* Both of these radical roots have been used extensively in fiery concoctions designed to bring comfort to sufferers of gout, rheumatism, sciatica and other non-specific aches and pains. It really is hair raising and although I am assured that it should be drunk I do wonder if it should be rubbed in instead! Take 50g(2oz) of fresh radish or horseradish root, unpeeled but washed, and chop finely. Place in 1 litre (1¾ pints) of white wine, seal and leave for approximately three weeks. Strain and drink a wineglassful twice a day before meals.

BRUISES

When we were children and had bruised ourselves the first thing that any well-meaning adult would do was to thrust the injured limb under cold water 'to bring out the bruise'. I am sure that this was intended to create such exquisite agony that we forgot the original injury. Icy cold water does have the effect of immediately, if temporarily, freezing the affected area and of relieving tension, pain and shock. It also reduces the swelling. However, a kinder method of treating bruising is to swab with a warm compress followed by a gentle massage with a healing oil to stimulate the circulation and prevent further discoloration. Warm poultices also stimulate the circulation whilst they heal and soothe

and are most frequently used on those horrendously painful bony parts of the body such as the shin which would, at one time, have been rubbed with a penny or wrapped in oak leaves. Another part of the body which is particularly vulnerable to bruising is the eye and anyone who has sported a spectacularly disastrous black eye will know that the remedies suggested vary from the awful application of extract of lead, which is not to be recommended, to the laying on of expensive raw steaks, slices of cucumber and ice bags.

People who bruise easily or excessively are often found to be deficient in vitamin C or to suffer from poor circulation in which case a change of diet might be advisable. Blows or bruising to the head may cause concussion.

Soothing Lotions and Poultices

● *Tincture of arnica* A few drops of tincture in a bowl of cold water is extremely effective. However, care should be taken as it can cause a rash on sensitive skin. Arnica must not be used undiluted or on broken skin.

● *Witch hazel* Cool and sweet smelling, this is a great favourite with children and can be used undiluted but as it is astringent it can cause a mild rash on sensitive skins.

● *Thyme or lavender vinegar* Both of these herbs are antiseptic and vinegar helps bruising to fade quickly.

● *Comfrey tea* Used either warm or cold on a compress comfrey has a great reputation as a healer of external injuries and is gentle enough to use on the eye.

● *Hyssop infusion* Known to be very beneficial in the healing of black eyes, both the fresh juice and the infusion of hyssop will reduce bruising quickly.

● *Onion juice* Half an onion rubbed on

a bruised area is quick, cheap, effective
– and antisocial.

• *Marjoram and honey* Four sprigs of
fresh or 1 teaspoon of dried marjoram,
pounded with a little vinegar then
mixed to a thick paste with honey is an
easy poultice to use on bruising and one
that children will love.

• *Parsley butter* This cook's remedy is
surprisingly effective.

• *Comfrey, feverfew or hyssop* A standard
poultice made with 1 tablespoon of the
dried herb to 300ml($\frac{1}{2}$ pint) of boiling
water applied warm to the affected area
and bandaged, if possible, heals bruising and eases pain. The fresh crushed
leaves of any one of these magical
herbs can be used with equally good
results.

• *Marigold heads* A standard poultice
made with dried marigold petals and
applied warm between two layers of
gauze is a soothing poultice for black
eyes.

• *Oatmeal or oats* Mixed to a thick
paste with boiling water, this is a stable
boy's remedy for bruised shins. Apply
on a cloth and bandage in place.

• *Lavender, hyssop or marjoram oils* Use
2 drops of the essential oil of any one of
these antiseptic and healing oils to 2
teaspoons of sunflower oil and rub
gently into the painful area.

• *Vitamin E oil* A little of this oil rubbed into a bruise will help it clear
quickly.

• *Marigold oil* Gentle and unperfumed marigold oil rapidly dissipates
bruises and blemishes on the face and
around the eyes.

Aches and Pains in the Head and Face

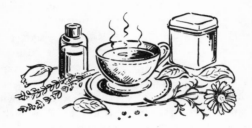

Headache

There are so many reasons for a head-ache, from the self-inflicted ghastliness of a hangover to the genuinely fearsome migraine (for which you may not have an answer), and these will be looked at under the relevant headings. There are early-morning headaches which can be caused by low blood sugar level and are eased by taking a spoonful of honey and there are those headaches which many adults suffer from and which are only cured with an injection of capital, but the majority have their cause in other physical conditions such as colds, catarrh, constipation, cystitis, poor digestion, fatigue, allergic reaction (particularly to food and smell), emo-tional dramas, period problems, aches and pains, a fall or concussion, high or low blood pressure, strain and tension, wisdom teeth and specific illnesses. The remedies found under those headings will hopefully relieve the condition and thus the headache. If you suddenly begin to suffer from persistent head-aches which have no understandable cause – eye strain, using a V.D.U. without an anti-glare shield, too much sun – take professional advice without hesitation. If you feel headachy and 'out of sorts' cut out the obvious nasties: smoking, tea, coffee, chocolate, cheese, milk, red wine, brandy. Drink instead lots of good, clear water, especially car-bonated mineral water.

In countries where too much sun is an ever-present problem a snake band around the head or worn as a hat band is still considered to have a function beyond the sartorial in keeping sun stroke and headaches at bay. If the cause of a headache is eye strain obviously one's eyes should be tested but sore eyes can also be the cause so bathe them morning and night with either eyebright or cold boiled water. The smell of certain flowers can cause headaches, especially lilac, madonna lilies, heliotrope and gardenia, and many of those perfumes which are predominantly musk or gardenia-based have the same effect.

Folklore tells us we should never smell poppies or sleep under the cypress for to do so will give us a pain in the head and lead to madness! However to wear a good bunch of lavender beneath our hats would certainly have ensured immunity, probably as a result of all those lovely antiseptic oils warming up and guarding us against infection. It would undoubtedly have looked and smelled better than the favourite cure for a headache which was the standard wrapping of vinegar and brown paper or the more esoteric combination of goat's dung and squill (vinegar of ammonia). Poultices were also mentioned frequently: slices of cucumber or raw potatoes laid on brow and temples to remedy sunstroke and headaches caused by sultry weather, houseleek leaves crushed and applied to hot and aching heads and a marvellous compress made of elder leaves crushed with salt which brings immediate relief but unfortunately smells vilely foetid. Ivy leaves are also reputed to ease a headache but counteract the good they do by causing a rash. Too numerous to mention are the herbal teas which will relieve the pain of an aching head but any which will relieve tension will help.

Sweet-Smelling Remedies

● *Scented leaves* Any deliciously scented leaf when rubbed between the fingers and inhaled deeply will clear the head and make you feel more alive. This is one of the reasons, I am sure, that cottage dwellers grew their most scented plants beside the kitchen door. The most effective are lemon verbena, lemon balm, dill, sage, peppermint, spearmint, rose, lavender and violet. The smell of hops will soothe whilst

cloves or the peel of oranges and lemons invigorate and an infusion of mint, sage or fennel or two tablespoons each of hop tea and vinegar can be inhaled or used on a cool compress.

● *A headache pillow from America* Mix together 50g(2oz) each of lavender, marjoram, rose petals, betony and rose leaf and 15g(½oz) of cloves. Sew them into a cotton case and keep it beneath your pillow.

● *Lavender vinegar* Herbal vinegars were considered disinfectant and those that were most frequently used in the sick room were rue and rosemary. Lavender vinegar will refresh and clear a thick head as well as being strongly antiseptic.

Lavender Water
2 tablespoons dried lavender
1 tablespoon dried sweet cicely
2 teaspoons cinnamon
1 nutmeg, grated
1 litre(1¾ pints) surgical spirit

Put all the ingredients together in a large jar. Seal with a non-metal lid and stand in a warm place for two weeks. Strain, bottle and seal. It makes a wonderfully spicy and aromatic lotion to use on a compress. Lavender water and eau de Cologne were great favourites amongst ladies of a certain age and could be dropped on to a handkerchief or carried in crystal form.

● *Rose* Essential oil of rose, that most tranquillizing of perfumes, added a few drops at a time to a warm bath or cool compress will bring exquisite relief.
● *Attar of roses* Cover a jar of fragrant red rose petals with pure alcohol (B.P. not gin). Leave to stand uncovered in the sun until all the perfume is in the liquid. Rub on the wrists and temples to fragrantly relieve an aching head.

• *Rose petal vinegar* Two tablespoons of rose petal vinegar added to 1 litre (1¾ pints) of water has a fragrant, refreshing smell which is very soothing. It is also invaluable as a face wash for a patient who is running a high fever. It eradicates the sour odour and helps to restore the acid balance of the skin thus preventing the scaly cracking, particularly of the lips, which often occurs after the disrupting heat of a fever. Mothers nursing small children will find it invaluable on their own harassed brows. Like all herb and flower vinegars, rose petal vinegar is very easy to make. Simply cram a wide-necked jar full of scented red rose petals, stand the jar on a thick cloth and very, very slowly fill it up with hot white malt vinegar. Do not fill too quickly for this will crack the glass. Seal with a non-metal lid and leave on a windowsill for two weeks, shaking every day.

• *Malt vinegar* Apart from the deliciously fragrant and therapeutic vinegars given above, plain malt vinegar can also have surprisingly beneficial effects. The fumes of hot vinegar can be inhaled, it can be used cold on a compress to place on the temples or it can be added to herbal tea instead of lemon to cure a headache.

• *Watercress vinegar* Boil 600ml(1 pint) of vinegar with a handful of watercress and leave to stand for two hours. Strain, bottle and keep refrigerated. Use as malt vinegar.

• *Massage oil* Massage to the back of the neck on either side of the spinal column, the temples and the scalp will ease tension tremendously, but one of the best ways of curing a thumping headache is to massage your feet or get someone else to do it for you. The particular area to work on is where the toes join the top of the foot. Knead and stroke gently and allow your mind to wander off somewhere else – you will find that this is truly amazing. For the best results massage with one of the following essential oils in a dilution of almond oil: peppermint, rosemary, cloves, aniseed, marigold oil for the temples; wintergreen for the back of the neck. Tiger balm can be popped into a handbag or pocket and taken anywhere for any emergency.

• *Lemon* Salted lemon juice or cut lemons applied to the temple are old-fashioned methods of easing the pain.

• *Basil leaves* These should be chewed.

• *Rosemary oil* Take a good handful of fresh rosemary leaves or 'needles'. Pound them with 1 tablespoon of olive oil using a pestle and mortar. Transfer this mixture to a wide-necked jar and fill up with 300ml(½ pint) of olive oil. Seal and leave in a warm place for two weeks then strain and rebottle. Rub on the temples when necessary. I use this mixture to baste lamb as well as to cure my headaches. Marigold oil can be made in the same way but using all the flower head.

• *Lavender oil* Take 3 drops on a cube of sugar to ease an aching head.

Soothing Teas

• *Violet, viper's bugloss, vervain, elderflower, camomile, lime, lavender, mignonette, valerian or marjoram tea* All these gentle, tranquillizing teas are reputed to ease a sore head.

• *Camomile, mint and catnip tea* One level teaspoon of each to 600ml(1 pint) of water will cure a sick headache.

• *Camomile and dandelion tea* Add a generous squeeze of lemon to a cup of this tea and take for kidney and digestive problems which are causing the type of headache usually associated with overindulgence.

• *Dandelion root* Simmer 25g(1oz) in 600ml(1 pint) of water for 15 minutes. Strained and drunk warm this has a detoxifying effect on the system.

• *Meadowsweet tea* The flowers and leaves contain the same salicin which is found in willow and which is a component of aspirin. How much more soothing and pleasant to simmer meadowsweet in water for 10 minutes and drink three cups daily to rid oneself of a clinging headache.

• *Indian tea* Take without milk but with the addition of 3 cloves.

MIGRAINE

For those unfortunate souls who suffer from migraine – the thumping, head-splitting, eye-closing, stomach-heaving variety which necessitates lying down in a dark room for as long as it takes for it to go away – hearing their agony referred to as a 'headache' brings murder to mind.

Migraine may have many causes. Some sources regard it as psychosomatic which is borne out by the slightly sneering references in old medical books to megrims, vapours and vertigo which less emancipated ladies of a different era resorted to when they did not wish to do that which they ought. Stress and nervous tension certainly contribute to the likelihood of migraine but more recently it has been suggested that it can be as a result of the liver functioning incorrectly, a poor diet, constipation, eye strain, hormonal imbalance, allergic reaction to certain foods or troublesome wisdom teeth. However, and despite the amount of investigation made into the causes, nobody has yet come up with a complete answer and despite the great number of people who suffer from it the uninformed will still

continue to believe that migraine is just another name for 'throwing a wobbly'.

There are, not unexpectedly, few old-fashioned suggestions for curing this type of malevolent headache and the most sensible advice is to lie down in a dark, cool, well-aired room, under plenty of warm covers and in utter quiet. If the migraine has not eased within 24 hours call in a professional to put you out of your agony. Follow the dietary advice given under **Constipation** and at the first signs drink lots of water to detoxify the system and reduce water retention which may be the cause. Try to relax and take a calming tea well sweetened with honey. Bathe the eyes with cold water and massage the head, working with the fingertips and starting at the back of the neck at a point on either side of the spinal column, going over the scalp in small circular movements until you can feel it relaxing, then coming down to the temples and to the corner of the jaw bone.

Quick Comforters

The following are suggestions for alleviating and preventing the pain of migraine getting any worse once the first nagging symptoms appear. Hopefully they will help you to relax and stop panicking. Some of the remedies given under **Headache** may also help.

• *Baked potato* Eat plain without salt, butter or cheese (cheese may be a contributory factor in migraine). This is one remedy which I find works very well indeed.

• *Tinned tomatoes* Simmer tinned tomatoes with lots of basil and serve with a dash of vinegar.

• *Fruit ice cubes* Made with lemon or pineapple juice, these can be sucked when drinks may cause nausea. The icy cubes are wonderfully soothing to sore throats and can also be given to feverish children but should then be frozen on sticks to prevent accidents.

• *Candied angelica* Chew small pieces regularly, but not just before going to bed as it could stop you sleeping.

• *Feverfew, betony, tansy, rosemary or lime flowers* Any one of these herbs may be made into a tea in the proportions of 25g(1oz) to 600ml(1 pint) of water and taken by the cup four times daily. Betony (wood betony) comes from the Celtic words 'ben' (head) and 'ton' (good). Therefore one can believe that a tea made from the dried plant will cure migraine. The dried powdered leaf can also be taken as snuff.

• *Vervain tea* This is an excellent tea to relieve premenstrual migraine.

• *Lavender* A mild infusion of lavender – ¼ teaspoon to ½ cup of boiling water – can be drunk regularly and lavender oil (see **Eczema**) rubbed into the temples will soothe and ease tension. Peppermint and lavender tea will help to reduce nausea whilst a poultice of the crushed, fresh leaves placed on the forehead will bring cooling relief.

• *Basil* Inhale the essential oil dropped on to boiling water or make basil tea.

• *Fennel* A vapour inhalant made by infusing 50g(2oz) fennel seeds in 1 litre (1¾ pints) of boiling water will relieve aching eyes and itchy eyelids. Bathe the forehead and temples with the cool liquid three times a day to relieve migraine.

• *Marigold infusion* Apply cold on the eyes and forehead.

• *Oregano* Use oregano rather than marjoram (the cultivated plant), as it is reputed to contain more thymol and is therefore more effective. The dried and powdered leaf can be used as a snuff to clear blocked sinuses whilst the fresh

leaf simmered in oil or lard is an old recipe for a headache ointment.

Oregano Ointment
50g(2oz) fresh oregano
250g(8oz) white petroleum jelly
(vaseline)

Place the oregano and petroleum jelly in a china bowl and stand it in a pan of boiling water. Simmer gently for one hour. Strain and press out through a fine cloth then pot and seal. This not only brings relief to an aching head when rubbed on the temples but will also ease the sinuses if rubbed around the nose.

• *Camomile or lemon grass* Two drops of the essential oil of either added to 2 teaspoons of sunflower oil should be rubbed into the temples.

• *Rosemary water* This is an equally effective but poor man's version of the famous Hungary water which when placed upon the forehead and temples was considered a sovereign treatment for migraine. Use the fresh, flowering tips of rosemary and follow the instructions for making either attar of roses or lavender water (page 20).

• *Boiling water* A doubtful cure for migraine caused by too much sun states that one should take a glass of water and stand in the sun with it placed upon the forehead. When the water starts to boil the pain will have passed away. So, I fear, will the patient.

NEURALGIA

This pain, associated with a damaged nerve, is most commonly felt as a shooting, stabbing pain which usually occurs in the face and head and is often thought to be the result of a head cold or bad tooth. Old wives would have insisted that washing the hair and not drying it properly, sitting with the head in a draught or not wearing a warm hood in windy weather all contributed to neuralgia and the most likely suggestions for easing this shocking pain were to apply a warm compress or poultice or to take an analgesic herbal tea. Most of the remedies given under **Aches and Pains** will bring considerable relief but if oil or liniment is to be used on the face ensure that it is suitable for delicate skin.

Soothing Teas, Comforters and Compresses

- *Analgesic herbal teas* A tea made with an analgesic herb or one which will relieve tension is worth trying before resorting to anything stronger. Basil and sage, lemon balm, meadowsweet, vervain, betony, red clover, feverfew, pennyroyal and hop are all to be recommended.
- *Hop and valerian tea* Infuse one tablespoon of hops with one scant teaspoon of valerian in 600ml(1 pint) of boiling water. One cup only should be taken each night.
- *Hop pillow* Hops can be put to excellent use stuffed into a small linen pillow and placed beneath the head at night. They will send you off into a good, relaxed sleep.
- *Oats* A thick poultice of porridge oats warms and soothes but is very messy even though it does leave the skin delightfully white. A better way of using oats is to eat them daily as they are reputed to reduce nervous tension which in itself may relate to neuralgia.
- *Crane's bill* Bathe with warm water and apply a hot compress to the painful area. A hot infusion of crane's bill (better known as herb Robert or wild geranium) is a very old remedy.
- *Betony* Make a lotion using this which, because its hairy roots resembled the head, had a great reputation as a healer of aches and pains in that area.
- *Vervain, hops or camomile flowers or camomile flowers mixed with poppy heads* Any of these applied as a hot compress to the aching part, were gentle and safe and a lot more aesthetically pleasing than warm pounded cabbage leaves or the soft side of banana skins laid on the skin – both of which, incidentally, do work surprisingly well.
- *Comfrey* This makes one of the best herbal compresses. Mix the ground root into a paste with warm water. It is especially useful if the pain is thought to be the result of a blow or knock.
- *Basil, vervain and wormwood* These three were boiled together and the hot liquid used in a compress was the definitive answer to neuralgia and migraine. It was certainly a lot safer than a sinister unguent of aconite and hog's grease.
- *Essential oils* After soothing the area with a warm compress rub in a fragrant essential oil, first diluted in sunflower oil, to relieve tension. Lemon balm (balm melissa) or rose are the most popular. If more stringent action is needed then Tiger balm is known to bring almost instantaneous relief.

HANGOVER

Having a hangover is one good reason for signing the pledge. You do not need advice as to why you have a hangover but remember next time you drink alcohol to take more water with it so as to avoid dehydration. Any drink pleasantly diluted will give you the impression of enjoying yourself without the ghastly after-effects. Drink white wine well dispersed with sparkling mineral or soda water and avoid red, brown and temptingly tawny drinks. Saccharine in mixers will speed up the absorption rate of alcohol by the body and the quinine in tonic water can make you feel very depressed, more so than gin alone. People who smoke feel worse the next day but people who do not smoke appear to drink more!

Alcohol in excess causes dehydration because it acts as a diuretic and it also creates acidity. We try to counteract this with antacids whereas, in reality, a 'hair of the dog' or a large glass of unsweetened orange or grapefruit juice is of greater assistance especially if it also injects a jolt of oxygen to the poor battered brain and soothes the stomach.

A word of comfort to those who suffer: it is rumoured that only the truly healthy feel the agonies of a hangover. There are many good and practical reasons why this should be so but nevertheless I find it a necessary consolation in my hour of need.

Preventative Measures

A bowl of plain, live yoghurt will 'arrest internal putrefaction, have antibiotic properties which restore normal internal equilibrium' and avert a hangover. It is certainly more pleasant to take a bowl of yoghurt prior to celebrating than a coffeecup of olive oil which I believe works admirably but which I have never had the courage to try.

'Cures' to Avoid

• *Coffee* Do not drink coffee as it is a diuretic and beyond the initial stimulus will make you feel terrible.
• *Aspirin* Do not take this as it irritates the stomach.
• *Opium or bryony* Do not resort to these old-fashioned favourites for they will give you a hangover of a quite different quality.

Recommended Cures

Have a good breakfast of yoghurt and honey well sprinkled with wheatgerm or oats or dry rye toast and orange juice. Orange juice replaces the vitamin C lost during your revelries and is even better if drunk with sparkling mineral water. Other good drinks include warm milk and honey, cold milk and carbonated mineral water, barley water, a pot of weak tea with 3 cloves brewed in it, peppermint tea and warm water with lemon juice or vinegar.

• *Yoghurt or porridge* Either will help considerably in settling the stomach and are preferable to black bread soaked in water, roast onions and snails, although onion soup does restore the equilibrium provided it is eaten after drinking but before sleeping.
• *Honey* This encourages the body to rid itself of alcohol and also tops up the blood sugar level which will help you wake up and feel human.
• *Oil of evening primrose* Several capsules taken first thing in the morning will make the world look a rosier place.

● *Peppermint* Try a few drops of peppermint cordial or oil of peppermint taken in hot water.

A Hair of the Dog

● *Buck's Fizz* Mix together lots of bubbly champagne and orange juice – 3 parts champagne to 1 of orange juice.
● *Black Velvet* A mixture of equal quantities of Guinness and champagne. Lager will also revive with its vitamins and fizz.

● *Bloody Mary* Combine one part vodka to 2 parts tomato juice with a dash of Worcestershire sauce or a spoonful of grated horseradish for sheer shock.
● *Port* Winning combinations include 1 part dark rum to 2 parts port and 1 part brandy to 2 parts port.
● *Prairie Oyster* This is a mixture of raw egg yolk, tomato ketchup, Worcestershire sauce, cayenne, chilli powder, vinegar and salt. If you can stomach it you are already on the road to recovery.

Mouth, Teeth and Gum Disorders

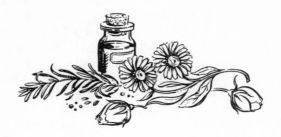

Toothache

'I told you so' is not the thing to say to a victim of toothache for they will already have perceived the point of oral hygiene and regular visits to the dentist and all they will wish is for the pain to be removed. Toothache appears to occur most frequently at night or during the holiday period, making the need for an instant panacea of paramount importance.

Sweets, sugary foods and fizzy drinks are appallingly detrimental to the care of teeth and gums. The acid and sugar combine to make the noxious plaque in which bacteria can fester and cause gum disease and tooth decay. A good diet from birth with the correct balance of vitamins and minerals is necessary for the development of strong teeth but even with the best possible advantages regular visits to the dentist are essential and so is regular cleaning of the teeth after each meal. Contrary to popular belief an apple is no substitute for this

routine, so if you cannot clean your teeth after meals buy one of the special chewing gums which dentists recommend as being better than nothing. Use dental floss and toothpicks (and use them gently) to remove small particles of food from between the teeth – this will do much to ensure healthy gums.

At one time toothbrushes and toothpaste were unheard of and the bark or twigs of shrubs were used with painstaking care to keep the teeth free of detritus. The end of the stick was chewed and softened until frayed and carefully infiltrated into every crevice in the mouth. Elder wood twigs were most commonly used in the British Isles but most countries throughout the world had their own favourites.

Considering that years ago the victim of toothache probably had to live with it until the tooth rotted in his head (the alternatives being too awful to contemplate), a great deal of thought was given to the best ways of preventing this happening. Appealing to Divine intervention was obviously thought the best method for the most powerful talisman one could carry around was the double jaw bone of a very ancient haddock – proving no doubt that you were a good Christian, knew of the haddock's Biblical connections and had no right to suffer the purgatory of toothache. Another merry thought was a religious script proclaiming one's desire to lead a good, toothache-free life, and this was carried around the neck for double indemnity. Rabbit's or sheep's teeth were also carried in a small leather bag near the throat or failing either of these amulets a hedgehog's skull or double hazelnut – which does not look unlike a large double tooth – were guarantee that should toothache strike the pain would be transferred to the charm. Another ancient rhyme suggests that one should chew the first fresh fern of the year as insurance against toothache and of this one would be guaranteed as it would have probably caused death instead.

It is interesting to note that although the majority of hare-brained superstitions were practised by the wealthy as well as the lowly it was the country folk who were the ones to employ sensible practices to keep their mouths healthy. They used elder toothpicks and elder vinegar as a mouthwash, they strengthened their gums by rubbing them with blackthorn or sage leaf and they made a variety of kitchen powders using soot, salt, charcoal, burnt bread or rye meal and herbs to cleanse and whiten the teeth at the same time as they stimulated the gums and disinfected the mouth.

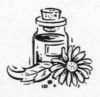

Preventative Measures to Take Today

● *Garlic* Take garlic perles daily. Rub the gums with garlic or pound a clove of garlic in vinegar and water and use as a mouthwash. All these are recommended to prevent gum disease and disorders but I would advocate following this treatment with a strong, clove-flavoured rinse to render you less antisocial.
● *Alfalfa tablets* These will strengthen the gums.
● *Vitamin E oil* Massaging the gums with vitamin E oil will both soothe and heal any soreness and keep the gums free from disease.
● *Eucalyptus oil* Massaging the gums with this is a very sensible method of keeping the gums strong and free from disease. An excellent mouthwash which will soothe sore gums can be made by bringing 15g($\frac{1}{2}$oz) of eucalyptus leaves slowly to the boil in 1 litre(1$\frac{3}{4}$ pints) of water. Simmer for five minutes, cover tightly and cool. Strain and add 2 drops each of oil of cloves and tincture of myrrh. Bottle, seal and keep refrigerated.
● *Blackthorn leaves* Infused in boiling water these make a gum-strengthening rinse. The juice from blackthorn leaves was reputed to harden the teeth in their sockets.
● *Lavender or rose water or mild infusions of aniseed, thyme, peppermint or marjoram* All of these are healing and refreshing mouthwashes.

Tooth Powders and Pastes

Leaving aside such mixtures as salt, onions, acacia leaves and other unmentionable ingredients which were favourites of the Egyptians, making and using your own tooth powders and pastes is safe and sensible.

● *Bicarbonate of soda* Being slightly abrasive, bicarbonate of soda will remove stains. Mix 2 tablespoons each of dried, finely ground lemon peel, bicarbonate of soda and fine sea salt. Pot and seal tightly.

● *Strawberries* Strawberry juice has been used to strengthen gums and remove stains. The following procedure seems a trifle long-winded but in reality only takes a few minutes and leaves the teeth truly clean and white, removes tartar and stains, soothes sore gums and ensures sweet-smelling breath. Pulverize 2 large strawberries and use the pulp on a soft brush to clean the teeth and gums. Dissolve 1 teaspoon of bicarbonate of soda in a cup of warm water and rinse the mouth well. Dust a little bicarbonate of soda on to the toothbrush and brush well. Rinse again with a cup of warm water to which you have added a few drops of tincture of myrrh (this helps strengthen the gums).

● *Gum myrrh* Five teaspoons mixed with 100g(4oz) of bicarbonate of soda strengthens the gums.

● *Cinnamon tooth powder for sensitive teeth* Take 2 tablespoons of cinnamon powder and 4 tablespoons of arrowroot. Mix together and store in an airtight container. Mix a small amount to a paste with water when needed. If the teeth are not too sensitive a pinch of salt may be added for extra cleansing power.

● *Salt* In an emergency salt can be used alone and is very effective. Rinse afterwards with a mild solution of hydrogen peroxide.

● *Orris root* As well as in cosmetics and talcums this powder has long been used in preparations for cleaning the teeth. The following recipe is very old-fashioned but the ingredients are

obtainable at herbalists and independent chemists.

Orris Root Tooth Powder
225g(8oz) precipitated chalk
15g(½oz) rice starch

Mix together and store in an airtight container.

Toothache Stopgaps

This is the point at which you have to visit the dentist unless you take the advice of one ancient medic who advocated henbane, in which case you will never visit one again (henbane is a poisonous plant). Another favourite was to throw the seeds of henbane on to a hot dish and inhale the vapours through the open mouth which I suspect was extremely narcotic and would put you out of your misery fairly sharply.

● *Cloves* The most popular remedy for toothache is to rub oil of cloves on to the gum around the aching tooth or to plug the cavity with cotton wool which has been saturated with the oil. Children with sore gums caused by teeth coming through or loosing their baby teeth will prefer it if the oil is mixed first with a few drops of almond oil. Chewing a clove on the aching tooth will also bring transitory relief – if you can bear the pressure. Oil of marjoram can be used instead of cloves.

● *Onion or garlic juice* Cotton wool soaked in either of these can be used to plug and disinfect the cavity.

● *Alcohol* Painting the gum with hot brandy, holding neat whisky or brandy in the mouth or plugging the tooth with cotton wool soaked in the alcohol all work well for adults.

● *Marsh mallow* A gentle and especially nice way of soothing sore gums and helping small children to cut their teeth is to buy the root(stick) and allow them to mumble on it. At one time the delicate pink flowers of marsh mallow were softened and chewed to ease aching gums and teeth but they are now so rare that this is no longer practical. What a pity that our native streams, where marsh mallow once grew freely, are so polluted by chemicals that we have had to resort to synthetic soothers.

● *Thyme or sage infusion* Place 1 teaspoon of either herb in 1 cup of boiling water. Cover and allow to infuse for 10 minutes. Hold in the mouth and swill it around well to reduce inflammation and infection when gums as well as teeth hurt.

● *Comforting warmth* Rather than placing a bag of hot salt on the cavity or poulticing the swollen jaw with tar as prescribed in days gone by, take refuge in applying hot flannels to the painful area or rest your aching face upon a pillow of warm hops which will have the effect of easing pain and making you deliciously drowsy.

CUTTING TEETH

Poor babies, how we suffer for them and how we suffer as a result of their restlessness, and there is very little we can do except apply a few harmless anodynes and lots of cuddles thereby making a rod for our own backs. All the signs of teething – a red cheek, fist to the mouth, tossing fretfully to seek relief from the irritation, incessant grizzling,

occasional upset tummy and frequently sleepless nights – distress even the most experienced mothers. Teething lasts for two years or so until the last of the milk teeth are through but it gets progressively easier as the child gets old enough to be able to chew on solids and can be distracted from twinges of irritation by play. Very rarely a mineral deficiency may make teething more prolonged and difficult than usual and if you feel this to be the case consult your Health Visitor. Resist the temptation to do as our great-grandmothers might have done and concoct a brew of poppy flowers and sugar to be given to your baby at night. It is too close to opium to be safe and by the same token 'knock-out drops' of any kind can be harmful and create a bad habit.

Gripe water is cooling, calming and safe for small babies and if it is rubbed on to the gum as well as given as a drink it will ease the irritation. Massaging the gum with a clean finger is a soothing diversion and cooled boiled water to drink will reduce the slight temperature that teething babies often run. Many mothers misinterpret the angry little fist being thrust into the mouth as hunger and react by giving a feed which will only add to the problem when the baby is sick or has a pain as a result of overfeeding. A little honey rubbed on to the gum will help the tooth come through more easily and once a baby is of an age to take solid food a sturdy piece of apple, carrot or cabbage stalk or a rusk of baked bread to mumble and chew on will help the process.

Very mild herbal teas are calming and will help a fractious infant sleep. Lemon balm, catnip, vervain and camomile are perfectly safe but to ensure that no muddle arises, buy a dried herb from a well-known and recommended source. Infuse 1 teaspoon in a cup of boiling water for 10 minutes then strain and give a dessertspoon either in a spoon or in a feeder. Toddlers can have up to 1 cupful. Mothers may require a little more.

WISDOM TEETH

See the remedies for **Migraine** and **Toothache** and visit your dentist. The pain from impacted wisdom teeth and the problems connected with their growth and position in the mouth are far-reaching.

SORE GUMS

There are several infections or diseases of the gums which cause them to become soft, sore or bleeding. Most gum disease is caused by a lack of oral hygiene where plaque has been allowed to build up, and around the teeth food has gathered in crevices and pockets of bacteria have built up and have burrowed away into the gum. Using a softly defunct or aggressively hard toothbrush does not improve matters: the former will not remove debris whilst the latter will cause the gums to bleed. Ill-fitting dentures can also cause terribly sore and ulcerated gums.

It was at one time thought that bleeding gums were a sign of vitamin C and B deficiency and a favourite remedy for this painful problem was to drink plenty of rose hip or blackcurrant leaf tea. Buy the rose hip tea and drink 1 cupful per day but blackcurrant leaf tea is easily made from your own 'catty' smelling bushes. Another 'catty' smelling plant which was considered to be the ultimate answer to bleeding gums was the modest herb Robert or crane's bill, a low-growing, pink-flowered plant

whose leaves change from green to red as the year progresses. Gums were rubbed thoroughly with the leaf or a decoction was made from it and used as a mouth rinse. Although I know that the herb has astringent constituents which will stop bleeding I cannot help but wonder if this remedy was suggested more to prevent gum disease spreading from one person to another for it certainly does pong and would alert the most smitten partner to the fact that there was a problem. Another leaf which was rubbed on to gums to heal and strengthen them was plantain which leaves a rich green stain, whilst elecampane, chewed to strengthen teeth which are loose in the gum, deposits a dirty yellow mark as a warning. However any of these herbs can be used as a mouthwash without dire consequence.

Other pleasant infusions to make and use as mouthwashes are bistort, marigold and agrimony.

For other soothing remedies see **Sore Mouths**.

MOUTH ULCERS

The small white spot on the inside of the cheek, the tongue or clustered on the inside of the lip was considered to appear as the direct result of telling a lie and as an antiseptic censure we had salt dabbed on it the moment it showed. That combined with a guilty conscience ensured that we kept our mouths shut on the subject. Ulcers are often caused by eating too much spicy or acidic food or as a result of stress – maybe that is where the superstition lies. They can also be caused by biting the inside of the cheek (another sign of tension) or a lack of vitamin B_2, which in itself can cause a person to become very twitchy. Avoid any foods which will exacerbate

31

the soreness and take garlic perles or chew whole garlic. Less antisocial remedies are to rub a few drops of oil of myrrh mixed with a little honey on to the sore spot or gently apply a little tincture of calendula. For further healing remedies see **Sore Mouths**.

COLD SORES

Officially known as *Herpes simplex*, these rather nasty clusters of tiny white sores on the inside of the lip easily gather and spread, forming a crust and becoming a 'bit of a mess'. Herpes spreads very quickly so take great care not to transfer the infection from your lips to your eyes. An open sore on the lip is not necessarily the only sign of herpes and in fact may not occur at all. You may have instead a furry tongue, red swollen gums and a high enough temperature to send you to bed, after which the virus will go to ground and reappear the moment you are feeling debilitated or if the lips become vulnerable after exposure to sun and wind. Herpes is a beastly, unsightly sore and has unfortunate and unfounded connotations which cause friends to recoil in horror. Zapp the blighter with tincture of myrrh or calendula, spirit of camphor B.P. or pure lemon juice. Apply it on cotton wool, which should then be burnt, and do not under any circumstances pick the scabs. For other remedies see **Sore Mouths**.

ORAL THRUSH

This is an inflammation which shows up as large, creamy white patches against the inflamed mucous membranes of the roof of the mouth, inside the cheeks and on the inside of the lips. Children are more susceptible to oral thrush than adults and it may be caused by antibiotics, allergies or too much sugar in the diet. Take garlic perles every day and eat plenty of plain live yoghurt. Rinse the mouth thoroughly with a strong solution of apple cider vinegar and warm water or use any of the mouth washes suggested for **Sore Throat** or **Sore Gums**.

SORE MOUTH

The following are healing remedies for sore mouths caused by a variety of ailments, whether **Cold Sores**, **Mouth Ulcers** or **Sore Gums**.

• *Lavender and honey* A few drops of essential oil of lavender in warm water to rub on the gums and rinse with is refreshing, perfumed and very antiseptic and will leave the whole mouth tingling. My favourite gargle and mouthwash for all throat and mouth infections is made by stirring 3 drops of essential oil of lavender into 1 teaspoon of clear honey and adding about $\frac{1}{4}$ cup of boiling water then diluting to a warm solution with cold water.
• *Sage tea* Boil 1 handful of fresh sage leaves in 1 litre($1\frac{3}{4}$ pints) of water for two minutes then infuse for a further five. Strain and add a few drops of tincture of myrrh. Rub the gums and rinse with the solution. This is especially effective if both mouth and throat are sore and ulcerated. One teaspoon of dried sage infused in a cup of boiling water makes a refreshing mouthwash but if a good pinch of dried ginger or cayenne is added it is doubly effective against *Herpes simplex* (cold sores).
• *Centaury* The leaves of this small pink-flowered plant of the gentian family which grows on our grassy cliffs

can be used to make a particularly good rinse for an ulcerated mouth.

• *Eucalyptus and clove oil* Disperse a few drops of each in warm water and use as a rinse.

• *Tincture of myrrh* A few drops in warm water swilled round the mouth hardens the gums.

• *Lemon, or glycerine and thymol* Disperse a little of either in warm water and use as a rinse.

• *Salt* 2 teaspoons of sea salt and 2 teaspoons of hydrogen peroxide in a large glass of warm water is effective. Hot salt water held in the mouth over a gumboil will help to disperse it rapidly. Rinse well afterwards with plenty of salt water to cleanse.

• *Sea kale* When we were children and in an attempt to make us eat the strong green leaves of curly kale we were told that it would keep our teeth strong. Sea kale, like cultivated kale, is full of minerals and vitamins and was often used as an infusion and mouthwash rather than as a vegetable, probably because it is rather bitter and harsh.

• *Black molasses, honey, garlic or vitamin E oil* Rub any of these on the gums to heal and harden but remember that sugary substances left in the mouth cause decay.

CHAPPED LIPS

Cracked, swollen or peeling lips are all incredibly painful and depressing conditions. At one time harvesters and fishermen knew these to be an occupational hazard but such soreness can be the result of many things. Weather can take its toll on the lips but so can running a temperature and illness. Sunburn, sunbathing, swimming in the sea and allergic reaction to food and plants all create the condition which may cause the lips to become swollen and shiny after which they will split or peel.

Always keep the lips well protected. When you are unwell keep them lubricated with white petroleum jelly (vaseline) at all times and especially at night. In earlier times butter or goose grease was used and was considered particularly effective if mixed with chickweed or marsh mallow. The gipsies swore by a healing paste of nettle tops simmered to a pulp and spread over the lips. Always ensure that a protective film of wax or oil covers the lips when you are pursuing outdoor activities especially water sports and sunbathing.

Lip Protectors

• *Emergency measures:* olive oil; castor oil; butter; a little honey mixed with rose water; zinc and castor oil cream; or lanolin. The last two remedies should only be used if you are certain that you do not suffer from an allergic reaction to either.

• *Marigold tea* This can be used cold to bathe sore lips.

Coconut Oil Balm for Burnt Lips
2 teaspoons grated beeswax
2 teaspoons coconut oil
1 teaspoon castor oil

Melt the beeswax and coconut oil together in a bowl in a bain-marie. Add the castor oil and stir well. Remove from the heat and pour into small jars.

• *Lip gloss* Put a ½ teaspoon of grated beeswax in a small basin with 2 tablespoons of cocoa butter. Place the basin in a saucepan containing a little water and heat until the wax has melted. Stir well and pot whilst warm.

Use at all times and at all ages to keep the lips protected.

Basic Lip Salve
2 teaspoons grated beeswax
4 teaspoons almond oil
1 teaspoon rose water

Melt the beeswax in a small bowl in a bain-marie then beat in the oil. Remove from the heat and stir in the warm rose water. Stir until the mixture cools and thickens. Pot whilst still warm.

This is an excellent everyday protective cream.

Minor Accidental Injuries

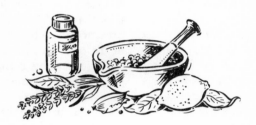

Cuts and Grazes

The old-fashioned panaceas given below are sympathetic healers for minor injuries. If, however, you are confronted with a deep cut or severe abrasion which is obviously causing excessive blood loss or needs stitches you should take the following steps. If a deep wound is pumping out blood this loss should be stemmed as much as is possible. Lie the patient down and raise the limb a little in order to ease the flow of blood. Remove, very carefully, any pieces of embedded debris such as glass. Do not probe further or attempt to clean the wound but cover it with a thick, clean wad of cotton and press it gently in place. Bandage firmly to keep up this pressure, adding more wadding and more bandage if the blood continues to flow. Take the victim to the Out Patient Department of your nearest hospital or, if he or she is not mobile, dial 999.

Hopefully the worst kind of injuries that you will have to deal with are those which an elderly friend used to dispel with the exclamation 'Goodness gracious, that certainly needs a sprinkling of magic dust', and out would come a small pot of golden powder, a mixture of flowers of sulphur and boracic powder, which she would scatter deftly over the well-washed graze or cut. It is important that the wound is washed with a mild antiseptic. Witch hazel, Friar's balsam or a few drops of tincture of calendula or hypericum in warm water will ensure that it heals without trouble. In an emergency warm soapy water, a few drops of lemon juice or a teaspoon of salt will work well but these are neither as gentle nor as magical as the herbal lotions and the telling of the tale that goes with them which fascinates a child and takes its mind off its woes. A gem of old fashioned 'sympathetic' medicine which children love is the custom of ritualistically cleaning the implement that caused the wound in order to ensure a good healing.

- *Garlic* Garlic ointment is one of the most healing unguents that you can use on open wounds. Garlic, pounded in water and applied on sphagnum moss, was an accepted field dressing during the First World War and garlic and honey pounded to a smooth poultice is still used to heal septic places, boils and ulcers.
- *Vitamin E oil* Used from a capsule straight on to a cut, graze or burn this works like magic.
- *Honey* Slapped on to a cut or graze and bandaged down firmly allows neither air nor moisture to penetrate and draws out dirt whilst it is healing.
- *Marigold, comfrey, horehound or elderflower* Infusions or tinctures of any of these may be used to gently cleanse cuts and grazes and an ointment made with any one of these herbs will also soothe and heal.
- *Poultices* Going by many strange names poultices were used to draw foreign bodies from a deep cut or wound, even gravel from a graze. The very best of these is the centre of the loaf, the soft bread crumb, mixed with egg yolk and warm milk and applied to any wound or to boils and whitlows where it appears to work wonders.
- *Parsley juice or fresh thick cream* Either pressed on to a wound and the dressing changed every 2 hours will ensure that a dirty place is cleansed most efficiently.
- *Other unusual but effective poultices* These included washing a wound with the water from boiled parsnips and then also applying the hot pulp. Crushed raw apples make a rather astringent application containing plenty of acid and pectin and no doubt heal wounds very well. One of the most pleasant smelling compresses for a minor graze is an infusion of southernwood which, so I am told, also brings relief to sufferers from frostbite. A marvellously warm and soothing mixture of thick slippery elm with eucalyptus oil is also effective on boils and whitlows. Less hygienic-sounding poultices used by wise women included fresh cow dung, puffball dust, horseradish roots, powdered grass, mouldy bread and butter, mutton fat and cobwebs. Knowing what we do today about penicillin, who can doubt their wisdom?

- *Compresses* The leaves of yarrow (*Achillen millefolium*) were used in a compress to staunch bleeding as they were in the days when Achilles made use of them to heal his companions' wounds. Other leafy goodies which might be used similarly are daisy, woundwort, marigold, green cabbage, plantain, nettle tops, alexanders (that gloriously green and shadowy relative of angelica) and golden rod.

Many of you may recall having seen the men in your family spit on a cut and stick a piece of cigarette paper on top of it to facilitate healing. I am assured that for a really deep cut a piece of old shag (tobacco) would have been thrust into the wound, a method of self-treatment which many sailors relied upon. Spit and rub has one advantage in that it can be used anywhere and it works, in a temporary fashion, as well as anything.

SPLINTERS

A sliver of wood, glass or metal, a thorn or a minute foreign object may manage to infiltrate itself beneath the skin, or worse, beneath the nail, and prove itself to be excruciatingly painful every time you touch it. If you are squeamish the best method of removing a wood splinter is to let the body take care of itself. The splinter will normally rise to the surface of the skin in a capsule of matter which can then be expelled with the use of a hot compress or a little pressure.

Those people who like to prise a splinter out with the aid of a needle should remember to immerse the area in hot water first and to use a sterile needle, applying copious amounts of an antiseptic ointment after the offending object has been removed. Safer by far for all types of splinters is to soak them well in very warm water and apply a 'drawing' ointment on a piece of cloth (comfrey is both drawing and healing). They will then either come out of their own accord or with very little pressure. For those beastly splinters which run down the nail immerse the finger or toe in a bread or linseed poultice or in fairly warm lard. Stubborn splinters may need a kaolin poultice to draw them to the surface but many will come out if a strip of sticking plaster is placed over them and left for a day or two. Warm tallow and resin was favoured by most housewives and is used even today in some households, whilst in some parts of the British Isles the sloughed skin of an adder is kept to wrap about a thorn splinter in the conviction that it has great drawing properties. It was also believed at one time that thorns caused septicaemia and would travel to the heart causing instantaneous death. Whilst we may now scoff at this it is not wise to neglect a splinter as it could, quite easily, become unpleasantly infected.

BITES

Snakes, scorpions and the bite of the madde dogge: according to physicians' manuals of two centuries or so ago these three dangers lurked at every corner and in Europe and further afield the chances of being mortally wounded in this way were undeniable. However, unless you are either very young, very old or of a weak disposition the bite of our only indigenous venomous snake, the adder, is not lethal although it can make you unpleasantly ill.

Wonderful stories of antidotes abound, such as serpent stones being boiled in milk and drunk. (A serpent stone was that supposedly created from the spittle of a ball of hibernating snakes.) Adder flesh and fat featuring highly in the list of fire-with-fire cures whilst bathing the bite in human urine was looked upon as a last resort. In Asia the juice and pulp from the roots of fennel were used to cure snake, scorpion and spider bites, a remedy in which I do not think I would have placed too much faith. I have even less faith in the theory that if you strew tarragon or coriander before you a snake will keep its distance and nor do I believe in the competence of ash plant and radish juice to do the same job.

Living as I do in an area where the adder is a fairly common sight I place my faith firmly in the belief that the snake is more scared of me than I am of it. I stamp my feet down firmly when I am walking and unless the snake is drowsing in a patch of unexpected sun it will be long gone by the time I arrive on the scene. However, if you do inadvertently tread on or touch an adder and it retaliates get to hospital immediately. The victim of a snake bite should be kept as still as possible during transportation. Dr Bach's Rescue Remedy (from health shops) will help to dispel the effects of shock but I do not really believe that the juice of honeysuckle, viper's bugloss or devil's bit will be an effective antidote. Lavender, however, is. In an emergency rub any bite or sting with bruised lavender and tie it down tightly on the wound until you reach help. The oil in the lavender is powerful enough to neutralize venom and will minimize the damage.

It is not too often that we are bitten by a dog but if we are it is usually pretty nasty. You should always go to the Out Patient Department of your local hospital for the wound to be cleaned and to receive a tetanus jab. Small nips from cats and dogs should be well washed with tincture of iodine or hypericum. Rabid dogs are another matter altogether and you should never ever touch or play with animals abroad, particularly in those countries where this foul disease is still rife. The cures given in old herbals are touchingly pathetic – eat the liver, well stewed in wine and syrup, of the dog that bit you or alternatively a brew of rue, treacle and garlic boiled in stale ale and rum taken for nine days to render a cure.

STINGS AND INSECT BITES

This group of accidental injury needs no introduction. When it happens to you, you know all about it and three things need to be clarified: what sort of insect? how can I ease the pain? how can I prevent it from happening again?

If you are ever in doubt about what has stung or bitten you, especially if you are abroad, seek immediate professional advice. If at any time there are signs of rapid and excessive inflammation, swelling or shock treat with Dr Bach's Rescue Remedy (see **Shock**) and seek professional help as some people have a serious adverse reaction to stings. Unidentified minor bites and stings can always be treated with ice-cold water or witch hazel.

Stings

• *Bee stings* Bee stings are nearly always caused by clumsiness on your part. Bees are not aggressive and because they usually leave their sting in you it results in their own death. Although they mean no harm this is of no consolation to you. Remove the sting with tweezers. Some people believe in sucking out the poison which is an acid and requires an alkali to neutralize it. Bicarbonate of soda mixed to a paste with water is the most effective treatment and parsley juice or honey will help to ease the irritation.

• *Wasp stings* The sting of the yellow peril is alkali and requires an acid antidote. Vinegar or lemon should do the trick although a more expensive suggestion is lean meat. Blue bags, which were used to bring whiteness to the household wash, were always applied to stings. Should you be so unfortunate as to swallow a wasp, an old-fashioned stopgap whilst you make for the nearest hospital is to swallow a teaspoon of salt. Wasps tend to be the most likely creatures to sting you in the mouth for they invade, without fear, the cup or food you are using. Any sting in the mouth can be alleviated with ice cubes.

• *Poison ivy sting* Wash the irritated area with warm soap and water and dab with calamine lotion.

• *Nettle sting* Rub with dock leaves or plantain. Alternatively drink nettle tea.

• *Jelly fish stings* Rub or scrape off the stings, which stick to the skin – you may have to use sand as the most convenient material to hand – and dab with calamine lotion. If you have been stung by a man of war jelly fish you should seek professional attention.

Bites

● *Ant bites* Sharp and sudden, these leave a small red mark and painful irritation. The formic acid needs cold water and bicarbonate of soda.
● *Flea bites* These leave a small red mark with a deeper red centre. Salt and vinegar, onion or lemon juice will stop the irritation. The old-fashioned cure for sand flea bites was to dab them with a little petrol but it is better to use surgical spirit.
● *Mosquito bites* Garlic rubbed neat on to the bite will prevent infection. In fact mosquitoes do not like the smell of garlic at all but if you draw the line at anointing yourself with the oil to keep them at bay eat plenty of the clove instead. Honey and baking soda stop the irritation and were the only treatment which managed to ease the miseries of the bite of the 'Blandford River fly'. Lemon juice or the rind of a lemon rubbed in well achieve the same objective.

Tincture of arnica, a strong infusion of feverfew, salt, eau de Cologne, gin, toilet waters or surgical spirit can all be pressed into use to relieve the dreadful 'itches' whilst calamine lotion is a very competent standby.

Essential oils of the following will relieve irritation if dabbed on neat: lavender, lemon (or lemongrass or citronella), eucalyptus, camomile and ylang ylang. They will also perfume the body with those fragrances repellant to mosquitoes and other insects if added to bath water or to an oil base with which to massage the skin. Insects may also be repelled from contact with human flesh by washing the body in a solution of 1 dessertspoon of Epsom salts in 1.5 litres(3 pints) of water.

In countries where the inhabitants suffer from mosquitoes they usually place nasty little killing devices on their windowsills. However, you may prefer to use cut onions or crushed garlic cloves instead, and remember that the smell of lavender also keeps insects at bay. Bouquets of tansy, feverfew, eucalyptus, lemon balm or elder will deter winged pests from entering the house.

Insect Repellant
½ cup fresh feverfew blossoms
1 cup sunflower oil
8 garlic cloves, well chopped

Simmer the feverfew blossoms in the oil for 20 minutes. Remove from the heat and when the mixture has cooled slightly add the garlic. Pour into a jar, seal and let stand on a warm windowsill for two weeks, shaking regularly every day. Strain before using as a deterrent or a remedy.

● *Bites from horse flies and unidentified nasties* Bites and stings from these can be soothed by garlic oil and bicarbonate of soda.

CHOKING

Choking is caused by an obstruction, usually food, stuck in the windpipe and affecting breathing. I have seen a desperate father hold a child upside down by its legs and shake vigorously to dislodge a 'gobstopper' and I have on occasion delivered the most mighty thwack between my own offspring's shoulder blades to achieve the same result. The accepted method, however, is as follows. Grasp the victim firmly around the waist from behind. Make your left hand into a fist and with the thumb extended inwards press into the middle of the rib cage. Place the right hand over the left and press sharply upwards and inwards into the abdomen two or three times.

CONCUSSION

Concussion usually follows a blow to the head and can be recognized by a headache or dizziness, tiredness, inability to concentrate or focus and a general malaise which may occur several days after the accident. A wrapping of vinegar and brown paper such as poor Jack endured may well have been the answer for a badly bruised crown, as it would have set rock solid, but I suspect that the combination of acetic acid and uric acid, which brown paper was at one time dyed with, must have had an overwhelmingly anaesthetizing effect and dampened Jack's high spirits considerably.

Practical first aid, however, tells us that head injuries should never be tightly compressed nor should one prod around to discover what may be broken. If you believe that there might be damage or if you suspect the jarring of the brain, known as concussion, you should consult a doctor immediately.

No Quick Answer

At one time daisy wine was considered to be the best possible tonic for patients convalescing from concussion but bed rest, warmth and keeping calm and quiet is the surest road to recovery.

● *Sweet-scented herbs* Orange blossom, rose and camomile pot pourri tucked into a small pillow or tied into a large handkerchief and placed beneath the sheet will ensure sweet dreams and a tranquil spirit.

● *Food for recovery* People suffering from concussion are rarely hungry. Therefore it is best to provide plenty of warm, nourishing drinks which are refreshing without being sickly and there are plenty to choose from within the pages of this book. When the appetite begins to improve encourage it with beef tea or a home-made tomato soup incorporating sage and basil, which not only tastes wonderful but is rich in vitamin C.

NOSEBLEED

Although a bleeding nose may be a sign of a vitamin deficiency or high blood pressure it is usually caused by a blow or overexcitement. It was, and still is, considered a safety valve and should therefore be allowed to continue unhindered for at least 10 minutes. By that time it should have expelled an obstruction or relieved pressure and the flow of blood should have diminished as a consequence of clotting. Do not blow the nose hard for at least 24 hours after a nosebleed as this might cause the blood clot which has formed to disperse and the bleeding to start all over again. If the nosebleed does not stop seek professional advice or visit the Out Patient Department of your local hospital where they will probably plug the nostril properly and also check on your general health.

The best and most comfortable way to sit when one has a nosebleed is on a hard chair with the head slumped forward, the nose being allowed to bleed into a bowl placed beneath it. To stop the bleeding pinch the soft parts of the nose together between finger and thumb whilst breathing slowly through the mouth. The popular remedy of tipping the head back and placing ice packs or cold compresses on the bridge of the nose is not a particularly good idea as it means that a lot of blood is swallowed, but a cold pack can be held on the nose or the back of the neck whilst the head is in a downward position.

Some people grind their fingers into their ears and clench their teeth whilst others leap into icy ponds in order to abate a nosebleed, but if it has not cleared within 10 minutes try plugging the nostrils with cotton wool dipped in lemon juice or witch hazel. A mixture of vinegar and water is also useful and although I prefer it soaked into a plug it can be sniffed up the nostril.

Other old-fashioned remedies included thrusting a cold key down the back of the neck, anointing the inside of the nostril with the styptic juice of periwinkle – which I advise most strongly against as it is potentially dangerous – drinking the juice of nettles or nettle tea, stuffing the nostrils with lady's bedstraw (this is not as silly as it sounds because the herb has such powerful coagulant properties that it was at one time used as an alternative to rennet to curdle milk), drinking whey and eating plums, both of which contain valuable vitamins and minerals. Grapes and raisins were other favourite foods to give to children who suffered from frequent nosebleeds.

A FISH BONE IN THE THROAT

This is quite a common accident but one which is nevertheless painful and can be frightening. Children and the elderly are those to whom it is most likely to occur either because they are eating too quickly and carelessly or because they may not be able to see clearly what is on their plate. In very rare cases the victim may have to be taken to the Out Patient Department of the local hospital but the bone usually dissolves or dislodges of its own accord.

Hints to Help it on its Way

Lemon juice drunk slowly will dissolve fish bones and a large chunk of dry bread, pudding or potato swallowed whole will dislodge an obstruction.

It was believed that the sharp point or edge of a bone could be sheathed with the fibrous leek and it was recommended that leeks should be eaten until such time had elapsed that the object would be passed out of the body.

Another very old-fashioned idea to prevent a sharp object which has been swallowed from doing any lasting harm is to soak cotton wool pellets in olive oil and to continue to feed them to the victim until you can get to the Out Patient Department of your nearest hospital. During this time you must not give the patient anything else to eat or drink.

Gargle with honey and cinnamon in hot water to soothe the scratched throat and avoid infection.

SHOCK

There are no pleasant, old-fashioned remedies for the condition of severe shock induced by injury or illness although it can be minimized by giving the patient Dr Bach's Rescue Remedy. The most important action that one can take is to summon professional help without delay and then to offer basic first aid and comfort. Lie the patient on the floor as flat as possible with the feet raised 15 centimetres(12 inches) from the ground, loosen any tight and restrictive clothing and cover with a blanket or coat to prevent heat loss from the body, but do not use an electric blanket or hot-water bottles to achieve this end. Do not give the patient anything to drink but keep him or her calm and provide constant reassurance and support until help arrives.

The worst case of shock that most of us have to contend with is that of a bad fright caused by a blow or fall or sometimes by bad news or an alarming experience. Although many of the symptoms may appear the same as severe shock – sweatiness, dizziness, feelings of nausea, thumping in the throat, shaking limbs and occasionally hysteria – the body will usually right itself without recourse to professional advice, although the ancient sages would have had us believe that cold water poured from a height upon the head of the victim or a sharp blow to the cheek would reduce an hysteric to normality.

Fright, particularly in the case of children and the elderly, causes distress often exacerbated by pain and anger. A hot drink will do much to restore the equilibrium and provide instant energy but do take care not to burn the patient's mouth. Do not fuss too much but remember that plenty of reassurance and lots of tender loving care will also help to bring the situation back to normal.

In the case of a fall or blow to the head seek professional advice immediately if the patient becomes drowsy or uncoordinated.

Sweet Restorers for Mild Shock

● *Honey* Added to a hot drink this is the greatest healer of them all.
● *Basil and sage tea* Half a teaspoon of dried basil and 1 teaspoon of dried sage to 300ml($\frac{1}{2}$ pint) of boiling water, sweetened with honey, makes a pleasant-tasting tea which induces a great feeling of well-being.
● *Orange blossom water and rose water* Orange blossom in hot water relieves anxiety, and the hands and face, clammy with fright, can be wiped with a cool cloth dampened with either of these refreshing and tranquillizing lotions. A few drops of the essential oils can also be added to a bowl of boiling water to be gently inhaled.

Burns, Scalds and Sunburn

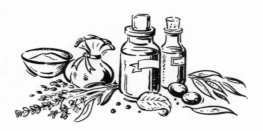

Burns and Scalds

Burns and scalds can be divided roughly into two categories. Those that are minimal are known as first degree burns, meaning that although the flesh has come into contact with either dry heat or, in the case of a scald, moist heat, the damage is fairly superficial although painful, and adequate first aid can be rendered at home. The second category is that of second and third degree burns in which a greater proportion of the body has been burned or a burn is deep enough to cause a wound.

The worst burns that most of us have to contend with are minor but nevertheless can become quite unpleasant unless correctly treated. Put the injured area into tepid water for a good few minutes to reduce the heat and relieve the pain. A few drops (up to 10) of tincture of calendula (marigold) or tincture of Hypericum (St John's wort) in a tumbler of warm water can be used to gently swab the burn. If the victim, particularly a child, is very upset camomile tea sweetened with a little honey will calm them and reduce the effects of shock and fright.

If the skin is broken the wound should be covered with a light, dry sterile dressing. Do not be tempted to prick blisters for to do so may cause infection. At a later stage, when it is quite clear that the skin is not broken, a gentle unguent may be smoothed on to relieve pain and irritation and to facilitate healing.

If the area of burn is more than 9 per cent of the body surface or the damage is obviously severe call for professional help immediately. Meanwhile follow these straightforward first aid procedures.

Immerse the area in cool or tepid water for at least 10 minutes. If the burning agent is corrosive (an acid) hold the burn under gently running water. If the burn is extensive wring out sheets in cool water and use them to cover the injured parts.

If the burning agent is a corrosive liquid, boiling oil or jam or a boiling, viscous liquid, cut away as much of the clothing as is possible but do not touch any material adhering to the burned areas—leave that to the experts.

Cover exposed areas with a light, dry sterile dressing. Do not under any circumstances dab with oil or powder.

Wrap the victim in a blanket. Keep them warm and try to get them to drink a little warm water to which a pinch of salt has been added as this will minimize the effects of shock.

If the patient is in a state of shock refer to the section on **Shock** for further first aid.

Keep calm and continue to reassure the patient until help arrives. Comfort and warmth are essential especially if the patient is a child.

Burns account for most household accidents and therefore equally numerous household remedies have come about which range from an ointment of sheep's suet and elder bark (elder was a very powerful 'fire' herb) to fish oil, sliced mushrooms and a nauseating nautical remedy of tar and mutton tallow. Usually, and not surprisingly, most popular first aid was to be found close at hand in the pantry: butter, lard, margarine, goose grease, eel fat, thick cream, sour milk, flour, starch, cabbage, potato, carrot. All of these remedies are based on quite sound commonsense because the most important priority is to neutralize the cause of the burn, to relieve the pain and to keep the air out, thus reducing the risk of infection, and lubricating the dried skin.

For burns caused by acid the old-fashioned remedy was a paste of bicarbonate of soda. For those kitchen minions who burned themselves clean-ing the ovens or making soap with the highly corrosive caustic soda there was the neutralizer of diluted vinegar followed by a covering of egg white. Scalds suffered in the kitchen were immediately covered with a dressing of boric acid powder and cotton wool. Burns caused by contact with lime were washed with vinegar and water then dressed with a poultice of chalk mixed to a paste with linseed oil, ingredients which would have been easily to hand in the workplace where a man might burn himself with lime. Linseed and lime water was another old-fashioned treatment from the same source. Peat soot and powdered charcoal are other country remedies which presumably found their way from the place of work, whilst some gardeners seem to have favoured a peach leaf applied smooth side down to heal the wound. Nasty burns seem to have been treated with a variety of vegetables, the most popular being poultices of raw grated carrot or potato or the leaves of cabbage cooked in milk. From the leaves of plantain in the South American jungles to garden cabbage in rural England the principles of folk medicine do not vary much.

Healing Poultices

- *Slippery elm* Mix the powdered bark with water and apply as a paste after soaking the burn in tepid water.
- *Yoghurt* This can be used to heal and cool.
- *Elderberries* A poultice of crushed elderberries is a very old-fashioned poultice. Even today the juice of elderberries is still used in parts of Europe to heal burns.
- *Dock leaves, elder leaves or comfrey* Mashed in butter, any one of these soothing herbs was used as a salve to heal bites, burns and rashes. The fol-

lowing remedy is more foolproof.

Comfrey and Honey Poultice
½ cup wheatgerm oil
½ cup clear honey
comfrey leaves

Whizz the honey and oil together in a blender until emulsified then add enough comfrey leaves to make a thick paste. Blend until smooth. Pot and store in the refrigerator.

● *Honey* This great healer can be used alone or pounded with marigold flowers to give a buttery golden salve.

Healing Oils and Infusions

● *Vitamin E oil* Available in either bottle or capsule form, this oil should be soothed on to burned areas. I have heard of several instances where people who have been most severely burned have used vitamin E oil directly on the damaged skin and taken large doses of vitamin E in conjunction with garlic perles to bring about such remarkable results that plastic surgery was no longer necessary, but I must stress that this was done under professional supervision. However, the results of using quite small quantities of vitamin E oil on burns and wounds are very heartening.
● *Olive oil, sunflower oil, pumpkin seed oil or wheatgerm oil* All of these will bring relief to a painful burn or scald and will improve the chances of healing without blister or scar.
● *Essential oils of lavender or peppermint* A few drops of either in a little vegetable oil will reduce the sting.
● *Liquid paraffin or white petroleum jelly (vaseline)* These will also ease the sting of a burn, keep out infection and reduce the risk of the skin cracking.

● *Marigold (calendula)* This cheerful golden pot herb which was one of the most widely used in popular cottage medicine has the least cooling look about it, yet the flowers pounded with olive or wheatgerm oil make an agreeably soothing and healing unguent for minor burns. A less sophisticated approach was to bind the injured part with the flower heads. Elderflowers were often used in the same way.
● *Garlic oil* Use this oil or garlic mashed well in one of the oils mentioned above to soothe and heal.
● *Comfrey ointment or oil* This is a sensible standby for emergencies.
● *St John's wort (hypericum)* This ancient herb was believed to repel demons. An infusion applied externally heals scalds, blisters and burns whilst either the ointment or the oil, both of which can be easily bought, are very healing salves. St John's balm (or red oil) features frequently in old herbals with instructions for dressing wounds. Cram 250g (8oz) of fresh flowers into a wide-necked jar and fill up with 500ml (18fl oz)of virgin olive oil. Cover with fine muslin tied down with string and leave on a sunny window sill to macerate for eight weeks, shaking frequently. Strain through fine muslin. The juice from the bruised or soaked flowers turns red upon exposure to the air and this 'red oil' was used to clean and dress wounds, but I believe that it would be preferable to use it purely to soothe.
● *Houseleek* Jove's beard or Jupiter's beard, depending upon your point of view, was believed to give protection to the home against fire and lightning. Should you be remiss enough to ban it from your roof and wall (where it likes to grow) it extends secondary relief to injuries caused by your improvidence. Use it as an infusion or warm poultice to take the heat out of burns. The juice

extracted from the fresh leaves and mixed in equal quantities with either white petroleum jelly (vaseline) or pure pork fat makes a soothing liniment for burns.

• *Cold Indian tea* This will bring instant relief when dabbed on burns and sunburn.

• *Infusion of elderflowers or camomile* Drunk, they will tranquillize. Applied on a soothing swab they will ease the sting of burns and sunburn.

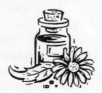

SUNBURN

Sunburn is caused by ultraviolet rays from the sun and can vary from the healthy golden tan which many of us hope to achieve to a nasty burnt blistering caused by excess exposure which is both painful and destructive. Not only does too much sun have an ageing effect upon the skin but it can also cause skin cancer, a circumstance to which fair-skinned freckled people seem to be particularly vulnerable. Our great-grandmothers would never have dreamed of exposing themselves to the sun as it would have been deemed not only inelegant and vulgar but also downright dangerous, for they took the threat of sunstroke very seriously indeed. Whereas today we will spend a fortune on sunblocking creams to ensure that we achieve a safe tan, they would have stayed beneath their parasols and hats and attacked the slightest reddening of the skin with hydrogen peroxide or a solution of weak ammonia!

Good advice is to take sunbathing in short bursts both before and after the heat of midday and to remember that salt water and strong winds will cause the skin to burn much more readily. Do not go to sleep in the sun, particularly if you are not accustomed to it, and do not allow children to become over-exposed. Most children have their own built-in warning device and become extremely tetchy when the sun is too strong or when they have had enough, so make sure that there is adequate shade provided for them as well as a good supply of tee shirts and sun hats. Sun-blocking creams should be used on holiday, particularly abroad and especially on children. Remember, the fairer the skin the higher the sun block number required to give protection. Rose water and glycerine will help moisturize and prevent the skin from drying out and although this does not provide a barrier it reduces the heat.

Contrary to popular belief – though it may have worked in the days when only a minimal portion of the anatomy was exposed to a fairly weak sun – spraying cold water on a hot body whilst sun tanning does not moisturize the skin. To prove the point try spraying cold water on meat roasting in a hot oven to see how quickly it will crisp up and become leathery.

Drink plenty of water to prevent dehydration and protect the skin, lips and hair before going to the beach. Take a cooling bath upon returning then anoint the face and body thoroughly with oil to keep the skin supple and smooth. It is very important to do this for children too.

Instant Relief

• *Calamine lotion* Alone it will reduce heat and soreness but it is very drying and may result in painful peeling. Use the following instead.

Calamine and Glycerin Lotion
5 tablespoons calamine lotion
6 tablespoons pure water
2 teaspoons glycerine

Shake together in a bottle and use at night when necessary. This is a very useful remedy to use on children who will sleep more comfortably after a soothing application.

• *Bicarbonate of soda or baking soda* Either of these kitchen standbys mixed to a paste with water will take the heat out of small burns. For all over relief from irritation add 2 tablespoons to a cool bath.

• *Cider vinegar or lavender vinegar* Add 150ml (¼ pint) of either to a bath. It will ease that prickling sensation and is also effectively antiseptic.

• *Camomile or marigold infusion* Add a good quantity of either infusion to the bath or use on a compress. Both herbs are also tremendously helpful in relieving feverishness in overwrought children when used as a weak tea or soaked into cloths and laid on the forehead or the back of the neck.

• *Aloe vera* The juice squeezed from the fresh leaf of the aloe and applied directly to a burn is gelatinous and soothing. (The plant will seal and grow again after such barbarous treatment.) It can also be squeezed out and mixed with cold cream, white petroleum jelly (vaseline) or oil to cover a larger area.

• *Houseleek* The old-fashioned method was to mix the expressed juice from the fleshy leaves with essential oil of rose, but just rubbing on the juice from the freshly cut leaf will soothe and heal. It was at one time believed that this remedy cured sunstroke when rubbed on forehead and temple.

• *Gin, lemon juice, milk, cold sage tea, cold Indian tea, eau de Cologne, infusions of nettle,* *lettuce leaf, camomile, comfrey or elder-flower* Any one of these applied on cotton wool will bring instant relief. Apart from the eau de Cologne it does no harm to drink some either.

Soothing Mixtures

• *Strawberries* Mash strawberries and buttermilk together to make a healing face mask. The strawberries alone will reduce redness and rash provided you are not allergic to them, and buttermilk is deliciously cool and minimizes irritation.

• *Cucumber* Cool cucumber sliced or mashed to a pulp makes a cooling moisturizer but an even better one is to blend the juice of a large cucumber with ½ teaspoon of glycerine. Keep refrigerated and use within three days. You can also dip slices of cucumber in pure lemon juice to lay on burns and 'hot places'.

• *Quince seeds* Soak quince seeds in water for two days. The resulting mucilaginous liquid soothes red, raw skin on face and hands. Windsurfers, sailors and skiers take note.

• *Yoghurt and rose water* Mix together 150ml (¼ pint) of plain yoghurt and 2 tablespoons of rosewater (elderflower water can be substituted for the rose water.) Apply where it hurts to soothe and cool. The application of this delicious mixture can be made into a terrific game to turn a cantankerous child's thoughts from misery to laughter. Rose water and glycerine, 4 tablespoons of each, is one of the best moisturizers for children's skin but it is not as healing as yoghurt.

Iodine Sunburn Lotion

6 tablespoons olive oil
3 tablespoons cider or lavender
vinegar
½ teaspoon iodine

Shake the ingredients together in a bottle and use when necessary. This old-fashioned remedy is antiseptic and healing.

Elderflower Lotion

5 tablespoons elderflower water
5 tablespoons glycerine
3 tablespoons witch hazel
1 tablespoon almond oil
1 tablespoon eau de Cologne
½ teaspoon borax

Shake all the ingredients together in a bottle and keep refrigerated. Shake well before using. This lotion can be used all over the body to soothe sun and wind-burn and is particularly useful to board sailors and water skiers.

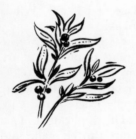

Sunshine Rescue Cream

2 tablespoons white petroleum jelly
(vaseline)
4 tablespoons anhydrous lanolin
1 tablespoon sunflower oil
1 tablespoon wheatgerm oil
3 drops vitamin E oil
3 drops vitamin A oil

Put the vaseline and lanolin into a bowl over boiling water and heat until they are both melted. Add the oils and beat well then remove from the heat and continue beating until cool. Pour into a clean pot and seal when cold. Use liberally on burnt noses, chins, shoulders and the like. Again this is a good cream for sportsmen who find that bony protruberances tend to catch more sun than other areas.

● *Pumpkin seed oil, sesame seed oil or olive oil* Any one of these used at night will keep the skin supple and soothe light burning.
● *Marigold and wheatgerm oil* Marigold flowers pounded in wheatgerm oil make a good healing salve.
● *Vitamin E oil* Applied neat to any burned area this will improve healing. It can also be mixed into white petroleum jelly to make it easier to cover a large area. If you cannot obtain the small bottles split open the capsules instead.

CHILDHOOD AILMENTS

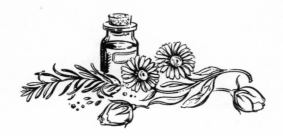

NAPPY RASH

Nappy rash may be caused by the chemicals and bacteria in the baby's urine and faeces but it can also be caused by detergents which may not have been fully rinsed out of nappies during washing. A combination or any one of these things can make a baby very uncomfortable. The patches of rough, red, occasionally raw-looking skin can be fairly localized or it can spread all over the buttocks, thighs and genitals. There are several simple ways in which you can ensure that your baby is comfortable and that nappy rash does not spread or become infected and thus heals as quickly as is possible.

Use terry towelling nappies with a muslin inlay and change nappies regularly and often. Always wipe the buttocks and genitals clean, then wash without soap and pat them really dry. If the baby already has a rash finish with a good covering of zinc and castor oil cream, vitamin E cream, E45 cream or a neutral white wax barrier cream. If there is no rash a dusting of baby talc is probably enough. Whenever possible leave the baby's bottom bare, which may mean frequently changing the undersheet but is worth it in the long run, and try not to use plastic pants more than is absolutely necessary.

Wash nappies very thoroughly. This means cleaning them, leaving them to soak in one of the antibacterial solutions made specifically for this purpose, boiling them well in a non-biological detergent or soap powder – do not use bleach – and making sure that they are rinsed in several changes of water. All of this ensures that any lurking microbes are well and truly finished with and that no harmful soap or detergent deposits are left in the nappy.

If after all these precautions have been taken your baby still has a rash look to a change of milk or baby food or if you are breast feeding ensure that the foods you are eating are not too spicy or acidic. Any radical changes to your baby's food and any persistent problems should always be mentioned to your health visitor at the baby clinic.

INFANT COLIC

Colic is not restricted to infants and horses. In adults it is called flatulence and is discussed under **Problems of Digestion**.

Babies over the age of three months occasionally suffer from colic, a sharp stabbing pain in the tummy which makes them cry quite uncontrollably and for no apparent reason, usually in the evenings. As most babies of this age are on a milk diet the most obvious reasons can be that they are being bottle fed and the milk does not agree with them, or that the hole in the bottle teat is too large thus causing gulps of air to be swallowed with the milk, or it is too small and the effort of sucking hard is tiring them before they are fully fed. If you are worried about your baby's health for any reason whatever make sure that you tell your health visitor or clinic.

Some people say that if the mother is on the gin or eats strongly flavoured foods, particularly dark green cabbage, this will affect her milk and give her baby a pain. Few people seem to really know the reason for infant colic although old wives and young doctors believe that an anxious new mother transmits her tensions to her baby thus creating a vicious circle of anxiety, alarm and anger on both sides. Our great-grandmothers, accustomed to large families and little help, would certainly have advised us not to fuss because the child will soon grow out of it. Paintings of idealised mother and child moments with baby stretched comfortably across mother's knee

whilst she tenderly rubs its back were not, I suspect, meant to be text book illustrations on how to ease infant colic but it is nevertheless the best possible method.

Sweet Soothers

- *Gripe water* This is the old-fashioned patent medicine for babies. Anxious mothers with indigestion should also take a large spoonful.
- *Warm water* One teaspoon of boiled water from the kettle will help.
- *Catmint or camomile tea* A mild weak tea made in the quantities of 1 teaspoon of either herb infused in 1 cup of boiling water is a very gentle and effective remedy for infant colic. Always remember to strain through a filter. Sweeten with a little honey if liked.
- *Fennel seeds* Older babies suffering from wind or colic will respond well to the liquid from ¼ teaspoon of fennel seeds boiled in a little milk for five minutes then strained.
- *Carrots and fennel* One carrot sliced with a small piece of fennel and cooked very gently until soft then strained and mixed with a little honey can be given to fractious infants who are starting to take solid foods.
- *Dill, fennel or caraway seeds* Infuse any of these three types of seed in the proportion of 1 tablespoon of seeds to 1 cup of boiling water. Leave to stand for 20 minutes then strain through a fine filter. Give 1 teaspoon from time to time until the pain eases. Dill seeds are an ingredient of gripe water which in some countries is also known as dill water.

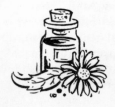

WHOOPING COUGH

Until recently whooping cough was one of the most prevalent and alarming of childhood illnesses, not only because of its immediate and unpleasant effects but because of the far-reaching consequences it could have upon children's health if they were not nursed and convalesced with care. It was not uncommon for youngsters to be left with damaged lungs and permanent vulnerability to infection. Small babies were and still are terribly at risk and if you have a child of school age in the same house as a baby and you know that whooping cough has been diagnosed in the area do your best to keep them separated. The first signs are a feverish cold and an unpleasant cough although the horrible whoop as they fight for air after a bout of violent coughing does not become apparent for about a week. Always seek professional advice.

It is apparent, by all the wise saws and saying which abound, that before the advent of antibiotics and immunisation a great many children contracted whooping cough. One which appears the most truthful even in our enlightened age is that if whooping cough starts in the bud of the year it will last ''til the leaves fall', or in other words if it has not gone before May it will stay throughout the summer and leave a child very vulnerable to infection for many years to come.

Because whooping cough is an illness which runs its course the wise women devised expedient methods of 'passing the buck'. For example one remedy suggested that the child should be passed several times through a blackberry bush and no sound must be uttered by any of the parties present. The lack of success was then blamed on any cries that the victim made when impaled upon the brambles. The same expediency applied to using the hairs from the head of a child who had never seen its father or from the back of a donkey with singular markings which when tied into a bag and carried around the neck would effect an instant cure. Other hairy nostrums carried about the throat were live spiders and caterpillars which, as they died a lingering death, took the disease away with them. Two further sovereign remedies were a powder of fried mice and onions, dried and nicely ground, or a syrup of molasses and rose gall – larva *et al*! The thought of taking either must have speedily sorted out any malingerers.

One particular old-fashioned remedy which I can just remember from my own childhood was to take the patient to breathe the fumes exuded from the local gas works. These arose from the lime used in the purifying process in the days of coal gas and were particularly noxious although we were all assured that to live in the environs was very healthy. The smell of tar – which I like – also appeared to do the trick and some people even went so far as to tie a tarry rope necklace about the patient's throat. Country children however fared far better than 'townies' for they were placed in a byre with cattle or sheep in order that they might inhale their moist, sweet breath – or maybe it was just that the calming presence of the contented beasts released them from fear and tension.

One of the worst aspects of whooping cough is the terrible panic that a small child can get into and which exacerbates the cough and makes it even more difficult for them to get their breath. All that you can do at this particular juncture is to sit them on your lap, leaving them plenty of space to breathe, hold-

51

ing a bowl in case they are sick and wiping the face with a cool, fragrant cloth whilst giving them calm, constant reassurance. A mildly sedative herbal tea taken with plenty of honey three or four times a day will help to keep them calm. Camomile is most helpful as it is anti-spasmodic and can be given to very small children. So can lemon balm and catnip – 1 teaspoon for very small children graduating to 1 tablespoon or 1 small cup for older children. Make sure that they take plenty of liquids to drink but not milk which can make them sick, although goat's milk is recommended during convalescence. Mare's milk was also thought to be very nourishing but is a little difficult to acquire nowadays! Do not give them dry food to eat as this will irritate the throat but make sure that they have a regular daily intake of vitamin C to combat infection.

Any of the cough syrups given under **Chest Infections**, **Catarrhal Infections** and **Bronchitis**, particularly garlic and honey, cabbage syrup or radish and honey, will help to ease the cough, whilst 'rubs' for the chest such as eucalyptus, essential oil of pine or cypress in almond oil, Olbas oil or garlic oil, together with many of the suggestions also to be found under **Chest Infections**, will ease the respiratory passages and make the child feel more comfortable.

Soothing Solutions

• *Thyme* Infuse 25g(1oz) of thyme in 600ml(1 pint) of boiling water, strain and take with honey: 1 tablespoon four times daily for older children and 1 teaspoon for babies. The same tea can be made with marjoram, mouse ear hawkweed (*Hieracium pilosella* which will reduce a fever), dried red clover flowers, lavender, honeysuckle flowers or elecampane which are all very mild and can be given as above to children of three years and upwards.

• *Lettuce* Simmer 1 cleaned head of lettuce in 600ml(1 pint) of water for 20 minutes. Drink the liquid three times a day.

• *Fizzy lemonade* This is helpful if drunk warm.

Onion and Honey Syrup
450g(1lb) onions
225g(8oz) garlic
600ml(1 pint) sunflower oil
150ml($\frac{1}{4}$ pint) honey

Peel and finely slice the onions and garlic and put them in a covered dish with the oil. Cook slowly in a low oven until very soft. Strain well and add the remaining ingredients. Bottle and cork. Shake before using. For children over two years old and up to four give 1 teaspoon three times daily. Increase the dose according to age. At one time 15g($\frac{1}{2}$oz) of paregoric (a medicine consisting of opium, benzoic acid, camphor and anise oil) would have been added.

• *Prickly pear syrup* Cut the leaves of 3 prickly pears into pieces (a feat in itself) and boil gently for half an hour. Strain and sweeten with unrefined sugar. Boil again until syrupy.

• *Grape juice* This is an excellent drink for sick children and it can also be used to great effect to cleanse the nose, throat and mouth.

• *Slippery elm* The powdered bark mixed with water and honey is both a food and a tonic.

- *Garlic* Try and get the child to inhale the volatile vapours of slices of garlic trapped in boiling water. Do not cover the heads of very small children as it may frighten them.
- *Camphor and naptha crystals* To hang these around the neck in a small, thick cotton bag is an age-old remedy.
- *Rum* Rub the back of the patient with old dark rum. Presumably the fumes alone are enough to induce sleep.

CHICKEN POX

In a society where smallpox took its toll of life and left its mark on many faces, scant regard was paid to those who got off lightly with chicken pox, an illness which would run its course and, unless you were very unfortunate, one from which you were unlikely to die. Apart from causing extreme discomfort this illness is not considered particularly serious unless it spreads to mouth and eyes which can be painful and may have worrying consequences. However professional advice should be sought when the first signs of chicken pox manifest themselves: the usual feverish shivers, runny nose, aches, pains and nausea which parents always associate with a child 'sickening for something'. After a few days the patient develops patches of flat red spots which become blisters and then break and crust over. This is the point at which they itch dreadfully and it is also the stage at which they will scar if they are 'topped' and spread disastrously. Very small children who cannot understand the consequences of scratching should have mittens tied over their hands. Keep the mouth, eyes and ears free from infection by using any of the eyebaths or mouth-washes mentioned in this book.

One treatment which all authorities,

ancient and modern, are agreed upon is that a diet should be followed which entails drinking plenty of fruit and vegetable juices. Lemon juice is considered to be the very best but a child with a spotty mouth will not take kindly to this and home-made lemonade or lemon barley water (see pages 126–7) would be better. Soft fruit juices – raspberry, blackberry and particularly rhubarb – are lovely and will be very thirst-quenching if added to carbonated mineral water. Rose hip syrup (page 73) is another old favourite and grape juice, like rhubarb juice, has been found to be especially beneficial. A great 'food drink' is the 'green cocktail' (page 77) which is a little too strong for most children but you could try them with a 'Sunset Slinger' of carrot and orange juice mixed straight from the blender.

A diet of salads, fresh fruit and lean meat or fish should be eaten in preference to anything else and carbohydrates, fatty foods and pulses should be left out of the diet until the child is well. Feverish children are rarely hungry anyhow so this should be no problem. Figs and molasses are recommended as being full of good things and the psychological advantages of eating stewed dried figs for breakfast was pointed out to me by one small boy who said, 'I like popping the fig pips between my teeth. It makes me feel better somehow.' A teaspoonful of olive oil, taken daily, will also speed recuperation. One of the advantages of having had chicken pox is that you will not catch it again.

Soothing Solu...

- *Witch hazel* Bat... in witch hazel. If ... ingly irritating wrin... liquid and use it to ...

- *Cider vinegar* Half a cup to a bath of warm water will relieve irritation.
- *Green pea water* So rarely do we get our hands on lovely fresh garden peas that this remedy comes into the area of luxury. However the water in which fresh peas have been cooked does relieve many irritations of the skin and was at one time used to soothe sufferers of scarlet fever. It also helps ease nettle rash and measles.
- *Calamine lotion or boracic powder* Either of these will help to dry up irritating patches but I think that this can sometimes make matters worse.
- *Nettle tops* Boiled down to a thick paste this old-fashioned gipsy method of healing pustules in and around the mouth also stops gums from bleeding.
- *Vitamin E oil* If the poor little victim is a young girl and she has some nasty scars left she will be devastated. Try a little vitamin E oil rubbed into each place as it is healing – I have known it to work wonders. Reassure her that in time the mark will stretch and fade away. Both parsley and garlic taken internally will also improve the condition of the skin.
- *Herbal teas* Sip a mild, healing, sedative tea such as camomile, basil, pennyroyal, marigold, vervain, catnip or lemon balm, several times a day with a little cinnamon, honey and lemon.

MEASLES

Although we in the West appear to take measles very much in our 20th century stride, merely calling in professional advice to confirm what we already think we know, it is a very nasty illness which can, if the patient is not properly [ca]red for, have unpleasant conse[quen]ces. As little as 50 years ago chil-

dren here died as a result of contracting pneumonia whilst suffering from measles and many children were also left with severely impaired eyesight or prone to constant ear infections.

The typical symptoms of measles are that for the first few days the child is listless and feverish with a cough, weepy eyes and runny nose, probably a headache, maybe tummy trouble and full of aches, pains and woes. After three or four days the temperature drops somewhat and they may have small white ulcers in the mouth. Following this they will feel feverish again and a red rash will appear behind the ears and across the forehead gradually manifesting itself over the whole body until they begin to resemble a boiled lobster. However the patient will probably begin to feel a little better as the temperature goes down yet again but quite often their eyes will still hurt and they may have ear-ache and a cough. If the last three symptoms persist and are painful make sure that your medical adviser knows of it.

The most important thing is to make sure that your child is warm and comfortable in a well-aired room and not subjected to full, glaring light, although I think that the days when we were kept in a darkened room are now past. Other children in close proximity to the patient will undoubtedly have caught the virus as it is at its most virulent during the first unidentified days of feeling unwell and also when the rash first appears, so if it does not get them the first time around it undoubtedly will by the second. As with all contagious illnesses a child who is run down, poorly nourished and does not get enough fresh air and exercise is going to be more vulnerable than a normally strong and healthy individual. The one consolation with measles is that once you have caught it you will never catch it again.

Drink and Diet

As with all feverish illnesses it is best to stick to a light diet of salads, fruit, lean meat and fish. Citrus fruit and drinks made from oranges and lemons provide both refreshing liquids and an extra boost of vitamin C to ensure a good recovery. One doctor I know of recommends a one-day diet of eating only grapes which has the triple benefit of eliminating toxins, providing valuable minerals and vitamins and cosseting the invalid, all of which will make them feel much happier.

Relieving Discomfort

See under **Nursing the Sick** for ways of making your unhappy child feel more comfortable. Apart from all the soothing suggestions given in that section bathing the rash with apple cider vinegar in warm water will reduce the desire to scratch whilst calamine lotion takes the heat out of the area and the water in which fresh peas have been cooked eases irritation. Massaging the chest and back with essential oils of eucalyptus, thyme or lavender diluted in sunflower oil or any one of the gentle 'rubs' suggested under **Chest Infections** will help to relieve a cough and tightness in the chest.

● *Eyes* These can be soothed with a mild boracic lotion – see under **Irritations of the Eye**. Once again however I cannot stress strongly enough the need for professional advice if there appears to be a problem with the eyes.
● *Ear-ache* This can be soothed with any of the gentle remedies given under **Ear-ache** but once again, if it becomes

very painful or persists, do not hesitate in seeking professional advice.
● *Gargles* Lavender and honey gargles will soothe a sore and irritated throat and so will any of the gentle, antiseptic mouthwashes and gargles to be found under **Sore Throat**.
● *Cough syrup* Ipecacuanha wine was the great standby of my grandmother's generation and although it is better not to suppress a cough there are some lovely mild herbal syrups mentioned under **Chest Infections** which will ease tightness and irritation.
● *Herbal tea to calm and soothe* Take 25g(1oz) each of the following fresh herbs or 15g(½oz) of the dried herb: balm melissa, elderflowers and marigold and 15g(½oz) of peppermint. Simmer gently in 1 litre(1¾ pints) of water for 15 minutes. Take by the small glassful three times a day. Other healing herbs with which to make a calming tea are red clover flowers, yarrow and vervain. Mother or father might require something a little stronger.

GERMAN MEASLES

German measles or rubella is not just a childhood ailment but one which adults can catch only too easily and sometimes with disastrous consequences. If a woman catches rubella during the first three months of pregnancy it can damage her unborn child. As a precaution all girl children should be vaccinated against rubella at the age of 13. If you have a child with German measles make sure that you tell all of your women friends who may have been in contact with you during the incubation phase and thereafter until the child is quite well. Unfortunately, and contrary to popular belief, you can catch German measles more than once.

The immediate signs to look out for are a sore throat, headache, a slight temperature and swollen glands. There may also be a slight rash behind the ears and then on the chest followed by a generally flushed appearance to the skin all over the body.

Treatment

Follow the advice given for **Measles**.

MUMPS

Mumps really needs no introduction. Adults can be dreadfully ill but children may suffer no more than if they had a severe bout of tonsillitis. The immediate symptoms are extreme tiredness, a sore throat, swelling at the front of the ear with the area becoming red and shiny (not to be confused with teething in toddlers) and then in the throat, usually one side swelling before the other. After this other glands in the body, particularly the ovaries in women and testicles in men, also swell which can be excruciating. There is a great deal of 'ho, ho, ho' about men catching mumps which is very unfair as it can make them extremely unwell and therefore they should know when they are coming into a household where children have the illness. Once again, contrary to popular belief, it is rare for mumps to cause sterility. Women who are pregnant can also be very ill if they catch the infection, so ensure that you tell all your friends. It is important to keep the patient isolated until you are sure that they are past the infectious point.

Like all these 'childhood ailments' mumps has to run its course and all that can be done is to seek professional advice and ensure that you keep the patient comfortable. We have all seen the classic cartoons of a swollen-faced victim with a cloth tied around the jaws, usually finishing up in a bow on top of the head. The old-fashioned method for bringing relief was to place flannel torn in strips over the swollen glands which probably did give a degree of warmth and protection but although a warm compress of arnica or tincture of calendula or a cloth saturated in warm St John's wort oil on the most painful area would be quite comforting, most patients prefer to be left firmly alone. They should be thankful that they did not live a century or so ago when they would have had their heads rubbed firmly upon the back of a passing pig so that their illness might be transferred to the unfortunate beast.

Comforters

Warm fomentations or compresses do help to ease the pain and a gentle application of essential oil of lavender or sage in a little sunflower oil rubbed into the neck and throat will certainly help children feel much better. Ensure that they drink plenty of water, fruit and vegetable juices but not orange or lemon juice – grape juice is a good alternative. It is unlikely that they will feel like eating although nourishing clear soups and fruit sorbets might be tolerated. It is also important to ensure that the patient does not become constipated and thus very uncomfortable.

• *Camomile and marsh mallow tea* Infuse 25g(1oz) of each of these flowers in 300ml($\frac{1}{2}$ pint) of boiling water. Leave until cool and serve with a pinch of either nutmeg, cinnamon or ginger and a good spoonful of honey.
• *Dandelion or nettle tea* Use 25g(1oz) of either to 600ml(1 pint) of boiling water.

Nursing the Sick

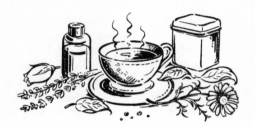

Fever

Fever or a very high temperature is the necessary manner in which the body rids itself of infection and as it is usually the result of an already diagnosed illness it should not be suppressed. If however there does not appear to be a reason for it occurring and particularly if the patient is a child, professional advice should be sought. As soon as it becomes apparent that a state of general malaise, loss of appetite, tummy trouble and aches and pains is progressing into a shivery fever the victim should be put to bed in a warm, well-aired room, covered with a lot of bed clothes, given well-covered hot water bottles to hug if necessary and left to sweat the infection out through the pores of the body.

'Breaking a fever' means helping a patient past the point at which their temperature reaches a peak and then drops, after which the body should be working towards recovery. During this time good nursing can achieve wonderful results and create a strong bond of confidence between patient and nurse. Caring for a sick person in the throes of a high fever can be a grim and frightening affair and in the past, without the reassuring presence of a doctor, it must have been truly appalling. Sponging the face and body of a patient with cool flannels, changing sweat-soaked bedclothes and nightwear when necessary, administering plenty of cooling sips of liquid and presenting a comforting appearance all do a great deal to aid recovery, especially in the case of a child in whom fever-induced hallucinations and nightmares can create terrible fears.

Cooling Lotions and Soothing Oils

Some of the least pleasant remedies suggested for 'breaking a fever' were to poultice the stomach well with a combination of onions and vinegar or to wrap a hefty bracelet of shepherd's purse, plantain and vinegar around the wrists.

Although bathing a patient in milk

used to be the recommended method of soothing and cooling an overheated body, much to be preferred is a 'blanket bath' with a soft sponge soaked in water perfumed with lavender or rose petal vinegar – vinegar will restore the pH balance to the skin and prevent it from irritating and flaking whilst the fragrance takes away the sour smell of feverishness. The water in which barley has been boiled was used in country districts and although it is a little sticky it does keep the skin smooth and cool.

The best lotion however is borage lotion which is made by simmering a good handful of the fresh, hairy leaves of borage in 1 litre(1¾ pints) of water for three minutes and then leaving it to stand until cool for a further 15 minutes. When it is strained it gives a lovely silky, soothing liquid to bathe a body with. The mucilageanous liquid also makes a very healing gargle and tea.

● *Foot massage* Rubbing the soles of the feet with lotus oil was the way in which the Pharaohs had their fevers eased but more prosaically and most aromatically rubbing the soles of the feet with a healing blend of essential oils in a carrier of almond oil will calm the patient a great deal. I always think that the feet are the keys to the soul and whenever I am unwell I find that I feel immeasurably better for having my feet massaged. The best combination of oils to use is a few drops each of thyme, eucalyptus, sage and lavender.

● *Lilac oil* When the patient's fever has abated but they are still full of aches and pains rub their afflicted limbs with this unguent which should be made in the early days of summer. Cram 100g(4oz) of the most headily scented fresh lilac blossoms you can find into a glass jar and fill with 600ml(1 pint) of

olive oil. Cover with a gauze or paper lid and leave on a windowsill to macerate in the warmth of the sun for two weeks or so. Press through a fine sieve and rebottle.

Potions to Reduce a Fever

● *Lilac leaves* An infusion of 1 teaspoon of lilac leaves in one cup of boiling water taken two or three times daily was a very ancient alternative to quinine in the cure of malarial, fever. Quinine was the old-fashioned standby for fever and is still used to prevent and remedy malaria, but before it was discovered the most commonly used country remedies included birch, ash bark, herb bennet, olive leaves, tincture of box and sorrel or purslane juice (the cooling green leaves of purslane were also laid upon the brow). These brews were taken at the first sign of those fevers which a patient might suffer from intermittently such as malaria and the following delicious infusion, which was frequently used in an effort to reduce the racking ague of malaria, can still be used today to ease the discomfort of a raging temperature.

● *Fever tea* Take 10g(½oz) of lavender and 5g(¼oz) each of heart's ease or pansy, borage, marigold and broom. Mix together and use 1 tablespoon to 1 cup of boiling water.

The bark of white willow and a tea made from meadowsweet were favourite tisanes to be taken in a crisis. Other healing 'fever teas' to be drunk at the first manifestations are elderflower, peppermint, catnip, lemon balm, vervain, yarrow and feverfew. Singly or mixed, as you prefer, all of these teas are soothing and will promote a certain amount of perspiration but nothing compared to the 'cold sweat' which breaks out at the very thought of the ancient remedy which extolls the virtues of powdered mint taken with the newly sloughed skin of an asp.

• *Hibiscus tea* This looks lovely and tastes delicious and older children will love a combination of rose hip tea and hibiscus tea (use the tea bags) which can be served warm or iced with lemon.

• *Basil tea* A tea made with 1 teaspoon of dried basil to 600ml(1 pint) of boiling water will be made more potent and pungent with the addition of the crushed seeds from 1 cardamom pod and ½ teaspoon each of ground cinnamon and brown sugar.

• *Blackcurrant leaf tea* Soak 50g(2oz) of the dried or fresh leaves in cold water for 1 hour then bring to the boil and infuse for 15 minutes. Take three or four cups a day.

• *Sage tea* When made by the following method sage tea has a slightly meaty taste and is excellent. Take 25g(1oz) of fresh sage leaves, 50g(2oz) of clear honey and 3 tablespoons of pure fresh lemon juice. Put all the ingredients into a heatproof container and cover with 1 litre(1¾ pints) of boiling water. Cover and leave to stand until quite cold. Strain and serve cold or reheated.

• *Gilly flower syrup* The gilly flower was the name given to any flower which had the scent of cloves, hence the confusion arising in old gardening manuals or herbals within whose pages pinks, carnations and wallflowers are to be found masquerading under the same title. The gilly flower referred to in this recipe however is the dark, dusky petalled pink perfumed with the heady fragrance of cloves. Take 100g(4oz) of petals and place them in a china bowl. Cover them with 750ml(1¼ pints) of boiling water, cover and leave to infuse for six hours. Press gently into a fine

sieve to extract all the perfumed water. Heat the liquid in a bain-marie adding unrefined cane sugar, a little at a time until the mixture has the consistency of syrup. Pour into dry sterilized jars and seal tightly. Take 1 tablespoon at a time to 1 cup of warm water or herbal tea.

Drink and Diet

When nursing a patient with a high fever one of the most important things to ensure is that they drink plenty in order to pass the infection out of their system. At the first ominous signs of an impending crisis administer lemon juice and honey or apple cider vinegar and honey diluted in plenty of warm water. A friend of mine from the Middle East drinks tamarind water made by soaking 25g(1oz) of tamarind pulp in 1 litre (1¾ pints) of boiling water for several hours. When strained it can be drunk by the ½ cup diluted with warm water. Taken every two hours or so it appears to refresh and to reduce temperature.

Lemon juice, lemon barley water, barley water, fresh unsweetened fruit juices especially pineapple and grape and a lot of good clear water, bottled if necessary, will all ensure a quick recovery. Very few feverish patients feel like eating but a few slices of fresh fruit or some grapes will usually prove acceptable.

Tiny Tots

Small children and babies can spring a raging temperature upon you without warning and it is usually as the result of an already diagnosed illness or teething troubles. Babies are very vulnerable so if you cannot identify the cause call for immediate professional advice.

Balm melissa, catnip, vervain and camomile tea, taken with a little honey and lemon juice on the tip of a spoon or in a small bottle, will help to calm a fractious child whilst plenty of warm fruit drinks or warm boiled water reduce thirst and aid recovery.

A few drops of essential oil of lavender or camomile can be dropped into warm water and used to wipe their hands and face which will make them more comfortable. When sponging infants down make sure that they are not in a draught and that they are dressed immediately afterwards. Do not leave a small child with a high temperature alone for any length of time.

Feeding a Fever

As has already been said nobody, especially children, wants to eat when they are ill with a high temperature but as they begin to feel better it is essential that they eat a little of those foods which are not only palatable but nourishing. The recipes below are easily swallowed and can also feed the rest of the family, if necessary, without them feeling that they are being palmed off with invalid food.

Oatmeal porridge and porridge oats contain vitamin B$_6$ and when made properly are very good for you. Porridge is a nice smooth breakfast food which is easier to eat than 'crispy crunchy corn thingummyjigs' despite any protestations to the contrary.

- *To make a true oatmeal porridge* Put 4 tablespoons of coarse oatmeal in a large basin and gradually add 300ml($\frac{1}{2}$ pint) of milk. Stir this briskly into 300ml($\frac{1}{2}$ pint) of boiling water and add a pinch of salt. Boil until it thickens, stirring continuously. Remove from the heat, cover and leave to stand for several minutes before serving with milk and honey or brown sugar.

- *Porridge using porridge oats* Use organic or conservation grade oats. Pour $\frac{1}{2}$ cup of oats and a pinch of salt into 1$\frac{1}{2}$ cups of water or milk, mixing well. Bring to the boil and simmer for five minutes, stirring occasionally. Cover and leave to stand for a moment or two before serving.

Beef Tea
450g(1lb) lean beef
pinch of salt
600ml(1 pint) water
pinch of mixed herbs

Shred the meat finely removing all skin and fat and put it into a basin with the salt, water and herbs. Cover tightly and leave to stand for one hour. Place the basin of meat in a saucepan in which there is enough water to come halfway up the sides of the bowl. Cover the saucepan tightly and cook slowly for three to four hours. Stir occasionally to ensure that the meat fibres are breaking up. Strain well through a fine sieve. Leave to get quite cold then remove the fat from the top. Reheat gently to serve. Beef tea is the traditional invalid food and tastes very pleasant.

Vegetable Soup
2 carrots
1 leek
1 onion
1 stick of celery
$\frac{1}{4}$ bulb fennel
1 clove garlic
1 tablespoon sunflower oil
1 bay leaf
1 pinch each thyme and sage
$\frac{1}{2}$ teaspoon sugar
1 litre(1$\frac{3}{4}$ pints) boiling water or stock
25g(1oz) flour
300ml($\frac{1}{2}$ pint) milk
salt and freshly ground black pepper

Clean, peel and dice the vegetables and garlic and put them in a pan with the oil. Cook for five minutes with the lid on, shaking occasionally to prevent burning. Add the herbs, sugar and boiling water or stock. Cover and simmer gently until the vegetables are just soft. Mix the flour to a smooth paste with the milk, stir it into the soup and boil for several minutes until the flour is cooked. Remove the bay leaf and season the soup well. It can then be either eaten as it is or strained and puréed to make a cream of vegetable soup or a cupful of the vegetables can be passed through a sieve and moistened with some of the liquid to make a very good meal for a baby (in which case omit the seasoning).

Chicken Broth
1 fresh free-range boiling chicken
1 onion, peeled and finely chopped
2 cloves of garlic, peeled and finely chopped
1 fresh bay leaf
sprigs of rosemary and thyme
1 litre($1\frac{3}{4}$ pints) water
25g(1oz) pearl barley
salt and freshly ground black pepper
grating of nutmeg

Wash the chicken and put it into a large saucepan with the finely chopped onions and garlic, the herbs and water. Cover and simmer for two hours or so. Remove the chicken from the pan and strain the cooking liquid into a clean saucepan. Dissect the chicken, discarding the skin and bones. Cut the flesh into small pieces and return it to the pan with the cooking liquid, barley and salt and pepper to taste. Simmer until the barley is cooked and the chicken tender. Season with the nutmeg and serve either as a broth or as a meat meal with potatoes and other vegetables.

Fillet of Plaice for a Child
1 plaice fillet
a little milk
salt
lemon juice

Grease a dinner plate with a little oil and lay the fish on it skin side down, adding a little milk to keep it moist. Place the plate over a saucepan of fast boiling water and cover it with either the saucepan lid or another plate. Steam until the plaice fillet is just soft. Remove from the heat. Take the fish from the skin, making sure that you remove any tiny bones – pass it through a sieve if the meal is for a very small child. Add a little of the milk that the fish has been cooked in, a pinch of salt and a small squeeze of lemon juice.

Tripe and Onions
450g(1lb) blanched tripe
2 onions, peeled and finely chopped
25g(1oz) flour
300ml($\frac{1}{2}$ pint) milk
salt and freshly ground black pepper

Leave the tripe to soak in a basin of cold water for an hour or so then place in a saucepan with enough cold water to cover. Bring to the boil. Remove the tripe, scrape away any rough pieces and cut into bite-sized chunks. (If you do not want an immediate revolution over the 'slipperiness' of tripe then it is important that you do cut it in to acceptable pieces.) Return it to the pan with 450ml($\frac{3}{4}$ pint) of water and the onions. Cover and simmer gently until the tripe is tender. Mix the flour and milk to a smooth paste and add to the pan, a little at a time, stirring well. Stir until the mixture comes to the boil and cook for a few minutes more. Season well with salt and pepper and serve with plain mashed potatoes or in a small bowl as a soup. Tripe, despite its elusive appeal, slips down the throat, is easily digested and is very good for you. It was one of the great favourite meals of my childhood and although the English frequently turn up their noses at it the French will pay a lot of money for the above dish, served in a *marmite*, browned on the top with croutons and a little cheese.

Baked Egg Custard
1 egg
150ml(¼ pint) lukewarm milk
1 teaspoon sugar
grating of nutmeg (optional)

Beat the egg into the milk, add the sugar and pour the mixture into a small buttered mould. Grate a little nutmeg on top and bake in a moderate oven until the custard has just set, or cover with buttered paper and cook in a steamer for about 20 minutes.

Arrowroot Blancmange
600ml(1 pint) milk
grated zest from 1 well-washed lemon
1 tablespoon arrowroot
1 rounded tablespoon sugar
pinch of salt

Put the milk in a saucepan with the lemon zest. Bring to the boil and remove from the heat. Cover and leave to get cold then strain. Put the milk back on to the heat and bring nearly to boiling point. Mix the arrowroot to a paste with a little cold water, pour enough of the hot milk into the paste to make it smooth then return it to the pan stirring continuously. Add the sugar and salt and let the mixture boil once. Pour into moulds. If you have the time you could make the blancmange even more tempting by decorating it with little faces made from lemon slices.

● *Orange tonic* Into a jug put 25g(1oz) of orange peel pared finely from well-washed oranges, 25g(1oz) camomile flowers and a few cloves. Cover with 600ml(1 pint) of boiling water. Allow to become quite cold and strain before using. Exquisitely refreshing.

BED SORES

Being 'bed-ridden' has problems which never even occur to the hale and hearty but remember how uncomfortable it has been when you have had to stay in bed for even a brief period of time. Recall how the base of the spine becomes numb, elbows and heels itch and the shoulder blades appear to have grown prongs upon which the weight of the torso is balanced. If you have to nurse a patient or an elderly person who is confined to bed it is essential that care is taken to ensure that those vulnerable points mentioned above do not become sore and in time degenerate into ulcerated patches, a condition which will be accelerated if bed clothes become moist through perspiration or urine. If small ulcers do appear you should seek professional advice.

Minimizing the Risks

Bed sheets should always be kept taut and free from crumbs and the patient should be carefully moved as frequently as possible. Don't drag the patient as this can cause tender skin to break. Try to lift them without damaging yourself. If you have to do this frequently over a prolonged period of time seek professional advice on how it should be done. Place a pillow between the patient's knees and ankles to relieve pressure and to stop them rubbing together. You can also buy sheepskin heel or elbow covers and undersheets which are comfortable if a little too warm.

● *Massage* Massaging limbs regularly will ensure that the circulation is improved thus avoiding the problem of cramp and it will be doubly effective if a few drops of essential oil of thyme, sage or lavender, diluted in an eggcupful of sunflower oil, are used. Some of the rubs suggested under **Cramp** are also very useful.

● *Rubbing alcohol* Gently rubbing the most vulnerable parts of the body with surgical spirit will minimize the risk of bed sores occurring. You could make up your own version of Hungary water to provide a really pleasant smelling and therapeutic version of rubbing alcohol. Pack a large jar with rosemary, lavender, sage, thyme and elderflowers and fill it up with surgical spirit or rubbing alcohol. Stand it on a warm windowsill, shake daily and leave to macerate for several weeks. Strain well through muslin before using.

● *Hypericum oil or calendula ointment* Either of these should be soothed into chapped skin whilst white petroleum jelly (vaseline) is equally useful on skin that has become dry and cracked.

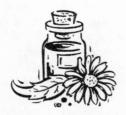

A HEALTHY ATMOSPHERE

To talk of keeping a sick room healthy may sound like a contradiction in terms but it is essential in order to stop the spread of infection.

The temporary hospitals on the front line of the First World War relied upon the use of lavender to disinfect and purify the air of their cramped and terrible wards and corridors whilst settlers in Australia used the leaves of the aptly named 'fever tree' or blue gum eucalyptus to achieve the same results. In truth, although the eucalyptus has wonderfully antiseptic properties it is rather the tree's thirsty ability to drain the mosquito-infested marshes and swamps of tropical regions that has most benefited mankind.

Fresh bunches of lavender or eucalyptus will sweeten the air and keep insects away but the most effective method is to keep a small pan of water to which you have added a handful of the crushed herb or leaf simmering on a hob in those rooms in which there is sickness. Not only does it disinfect but it creates a lovely atmosphere far more pleasant than that achieved with commercial sprays. The Greeks and Romans burned their herbs and spices in censers, keeping them in their rooms and carrying them in the streets to ward off infection. Myrrh, frankincense and balsam were popular spices then as were the other Oriental favourites, musk and sandalwood. The smell was probably very similar to joss sticks which are still lit in many households as a happy alternative to air fresheners.

Dried herbs – rosemary, eucalyptus, thyme, lavender, southernwood – crushed and placed in small linen pillow cases also sweeten a sickbed and help promote a good and wholesome sleep, whilst bay leaves and lavender were laid beneath the mattress in a house of sickness more as a deterrent to fleas and bed bugs than to cure illness.

Southernwood, wormwood, rue and elder leaves are other herby bunches to hang around the house. Elder leaves will certainly keep flies away as will the fragrant leaves of lemon balm, whilst rue and wormwood were carried in less than fragrant posies throughout the courts of an older and dirtier Europe to prevent infection from prisons polluting the air around the judiciary. The long leafy branches of the ash were also cut and hung around the house in the belief that they contained germ-killing properties whilst a bunch of ash keys (the fruits) hung above a baby's cradle ensured that evil was kept away and that the infant would thrive.

Hyssop and woodruff as well as meadowsweet and lady's bedstraw were strewing herbs used to keep the air in rooms sweet and healthy.

Not all plants had such benevolent properties for the belief that may or hawthorn brought into a house will bring bad luck (and bad luck usually meant illness) is universal whilst in Dorset bergamot over the doorstep portends sickness and death.

Burning and Simmering Herbs and Spices

At the time of the great plague recommendations were given to the wealthy to lay upon a pan of burning coals bay,

cedar or juniper, lavender and rosemary and to stand this aromatic burner in the central room of the house to fumigate and sweeten the air. More easily you can take a heavy cast iron frying pan and set to burn in it a minute amount of charcoal upon which you then scatter dried herbs, seeds, roots or powders. Alternatively place your selection in a pan held over a high flame. When they start to smell more pungent remove the pan from the heat and carry from room to room. The same method of strewing powerfully scented herbs on an open, slow-burning fire can be used outdoors to keep midges and flies away.

Incense Powder
3 teaspoons powdered frankincense
2 teaspoons powdered orris root
1 teaspoon powdered cloves
1 teaspoon fine sandalwood chips
1–2 drops essential oil of bergamot

Mix all the dry ingredients together with one or two drops of the oil then leave in an airtight box in a cool, dry place to mature for two months. When required sprinkle a little on a hot pan of charcoal as suggested above. The fragrance is powerful and heady.

● *Home-made joss sticks* Strip long stems of dried lavender and stick them into a convenient holder such as the soil of a houseplant. Light the end and let them smoulder fragrantly.
● *Simmering herbs* Another fragrant idea is to take a good handful of fresh herbs or 1 heaped tablespoon of dried herbs and bring them to the boil in a small saucepan with 600ml(1 pint) of water. Thereafter leave to simmer uncovered over a low flame. Top up with a little more water from time to time until the herb loses its pungency. I use a small night light beneath a fondue

stand to keep a pan simmering gently all day.

Stopping Infection Spreading

Medieval mothers may have scattered holly water from a holly wood bowl or cut a briar cross and hung it on the door to keep a house free from fevers whilst more recently lye (water made alkaline with wood ashes) and carbolic served to scrub every corner and surface in a dwelling. Today we ensure that a strong, pleasant-smelling disinfectant is used to wipe door handles, lavatory seats, taps and other areas which might harbour germs. One of the quickest ways for germs to spread is caused by our polite habit of covering our mouths with our hands when we sneeze or cough after which we pick up or touch objects in the house or shake our friends by the hand and pass our bugs straight on. Always cough or sneeze straight into a handkerchief which can, if it is linen, be washed in boiling disinfected water or, in the case of tissue, be immediately burned – not thrown into a waste paper basket.

Four robbers vinegar, not the pleasant variety made with fragrant herbs but a far more businesslike solution of garlic and camphor infused in vinegar, was at one time carried with one, sprinkled on a cloth and held to the mouth or used to wipe any suspect surface when one unexpectedly came into contact with the sick. Camphor, turpentine and spirits of wine were also incorporated into a 'bug killer' to be shaken into every nook and cranny where one sat, which must have made a

visit to a place of entertainment something of an experience.

Humorous though the idea may sound the juice of onions and garlic or the water or vinegar in which they had been boiled or macerated were used as very powerful bactericides which could still be used today except for the perfume which leaves much to be desired. Perhaps it was this very odour which also provoked their reputation of scaring off snakes and witches.

● *Oil of lavender* A few drops mixed into liquid furniture polish or a little almond oil can be used on those wooden surfaces which you would rather not clean with disinfectant and it does make the house smell delightful.

● *Fly papers* Flies are irritating and dirty but many people consider commercial fly papers to be even more unpleasant so make your own by spreading strips of paper thinly with molasses to which you can add a little essential oil of pine, although the stickiness alone is enough to attract and entrap them.

● *Eucalyptus spray* Put 1 teaspoon of eucalyptus oil B.P. and 10 drops each of essential oil of lavender and lemon balm into 1 litre($1\frac{3}{4}$ pints) of cold water. Pour into a spray container and shake well. This is a good pleasant-smelling, antiseptic solution to squirt liberally about the house. It also discourages those nasty pests which attack house plants.

● *Lavender and sweet cicely water* Use on a damp cloth to cool a fevered brow and hot hands and to wipe surfaces. See page 20 for the recipe.

ALLERGIES

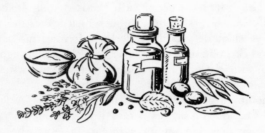

ALLERGIC REACTIONS

For specific problems see **Asthma**, **Hayfever** and **Eczema**.

From a layman's point of view allergic reactions can be put into three categories.

Contact with external or outside irritants (such as smoke, dust, feathers, animal hair, pollen, plants, mould or damp, powders and oils used in cosmetics, chemicals in hair preparations, synthetic perfumes, washing and cleansing products, air fresheners, disinfectants and the whole vast mess of chemical and synthetic pollutants in the air) can cause wheezing, sneezing, rashes, running nose and soreness, irritation and inflammation of the eyes, nose, throat and mouth.

Any substance which is ingested may set up an unpleasant reaction. Shellfish, fish, pork, nuts, dairy products, eggs, strawberries, tomatoes, white flour, yeast, artificial sweeteners, flavour enhancers, colourings and preservatives are all common offenders. Some people

are also allergic to antibiotics. The reaction to any of these substances can either be unpleasantly swift or make its presence felt after some time by causing sickness, diarrhoea, flatulence, heartburn, giddiness, sweating, skin irritation, headache or sore mouth and throat.

The third category of allergies is that in which anxiety, emotional upsets, stress, nervousness and illness can create any of the reactions in the above groups.

Allergic reactions in the first two groups are usually identifiable, ensuring that care is taken to avoid those things which will create problems, but the third self-inflicted group requires a certain amount of self-examination.

Emotional upheavals can cause the most devastating wheezes which in some circumstances may develop into asthma. This seems to be a case of adding insult to injury. When we are adult we can attempt to be more phlegmatic about our problems and in analyzing them overcome our fears.

Children, however, can rarely do this and they unfortunately seem to suffer in proportionately higher numbers than adults from emotionally induced asthma. Try to avoid letting them get into this state. Although it may be difficult when you yourself are under stress try to ensure that children are not embroiled in your problems. When you think that they may have a problem persuade them to talk about it and listen carefully to all that they say and note what they do not say. Be calm, practical and understanding, hopefully coming up with a few positive suggestions. None of this is very easy to achieve but it is nevertheless easier in the long run than having a child ill with recurring asthma attacks. Emotionally induced asthma in both adults and children usually becomes less frequent with the passing of time and ultimately disappears.

The way to test for a true allergic reaction on the skin is to place a small amount of the suspect substance on the soft flesh of the inner arm just below the elbow, cover it with a piece of non-allergenic plaster and leave for 24 hours. If the result is a nasty red pimply rash you have an adverse reaction. This test also works for some foodstuffs, for example strawberries.

Minimizing the Risks

Ensure that a sufficient quantity of vitamin B complex is taken daily and that food rich in calcium and magnesium is a regular part of the diet. Avoid of course those foods which you believe to be harmful to you, which are fattening or which have a bad effect on the skin, all of which can create further unhappiness and stress. Eat lots of fresh green vegetables and drink plenty of fresh water. Cut down on alcohol, tea, coffee, white sugar and salt. Practise deep breathing and take plenty of exercise out in the fresh air. Have more early nights, read fewer newspapers and watch a little less television, especially those doomwatch documentaries which are guaranteed to raise anxiety to a high level.

Avoid commercially prepared foods and more especially do not give them to babies unless it states most specifically that they do not contain artificial additives. Small children's and older babies' meals are simple to prepare yourself and whilst they may not be so apparently hygienic as commercial brands are more nourishing and tasty. Children do develop their own immunity to everyday bugs.

Do not use artificial air purifiers and sprays. Insteads burn herbs and spices. Buy or make wax polish and buy unperfumed soaps.

Preventions and Cures

It has been recognized for many centuries that honey has curative properties that verge on the miraculous and consequently much mythology and mystery has grown up around the beehive. Sufferers from hayfever and asthma were at one time subjected to a carefully controlled course of bee stings in the belief that this would bring relief from their misery. A less painful 'cure' has now been evolved with the discovery that for centuries beekeepers throughout the world have eaten the combs from their hives and recommended the practice to their neighbours to ease those ailments connected with the chest, nose and throat. There has been much research into the subject and several theories have been put forward, one of which suggests that the bee stings its own comb during production and therefore the all-important cure is in the composition of the sting. The other and more readily accepted suggestion is that those small neat waxy compartments contain not only nectar and honey but also large amounts of raw pollen. It would therefore follow that a greater immunity to a pollen reaction can be built up by eating the pollen-laden combs. To a lesser degree a preventative spoonful of honey or ¼ teaspoon of pollen granules taken early each morning should have the same effect.

Seaside dwellers will swear that a daily plunge into the sea or washing the face with sea water each morning will reduce the chances of affliction. Other masochistic cures include a cold shower daily and sniffing cold water up the nostrils at the start of the day.

• *Garlic perles* Taken daily these provide a more social antidote than raw garlic.
• *Camomile and sage tea* Both herbs invoke feelings of stoicism and calm.
• *Camomile, cornflower, eyebright or marigold* Use an infusion of any one of these healing herbs to bathe sore, irritating eyes. This remedy is especially useful if the eyes have proved allergic to a brand of cosmetic. If a tendency to allergy exists use almond oil to remove eye make-up as it does an excellent job while being very soothing.
• *Camomile tea bags* Used cold, tea bags reduce under-eye puffiness.
• *Lime, mallow and camomile tea* Use leaves and flowers, 15g(½oz) of each herb, boiled in 1 litre(1¾ pints) of water for 5 minutes. Strain and leave until cold then apply on cotton wool pads to restore brightness to red, itchy eyes. It is also a pleasant and soothing tea taken with lemon and honey.

Basic Herbal Moisturizer
or Cream
2 teaspoons grated beeswax
1 teaspoon emulsifying wax
5 teaspoons almond or sunflower oil
4 tablespoons purified water

Place the waxes and oil in a bowl over a pan of simmering water and heat until the waxes are melted. Warm the water and beat it slowly into the oily mixture. Remove from the heat and continue beating until the cream has cooled and emulsified. Pour into clean, dry containers, seal and keep refrigerated.

To this recipe and method you may add any herbal infusion of your own choosing for a specific skin problem. Merely substitute for the purified water a strong herbal infusion. For example 4 tablespoons of a strong infusion of golden rod used instead of water in this recipe will soothe a skin irritated by an allergic reaction.

• *Quince* The sharp, sweet spiciness of quince combined with honey and lemon has a gratifyingly swift effect on tickly throats, nipping in the bud any further desire to sneeze or cough. Below is an Italian recipe which, using the true quince, has a gloriously pervasive smell.

Quince Syrup
350g(12oz) quinces
600ml(1 pint) water
juice of 1 large lemon
clear honey

Wash the quinces and cut into small pieces without peeling or coring. Put into a stainless steel pan with the water, cover and cook gently until quite soft, adding more water if necessary. Turn the cooked fruit into a clean muslin jelly bag and leave to drain overnight into a china bowl. The next day measure the juice gained and add an equal quantity of honey. Bring slowly to the boil and continue on a slow bubble until the mixture is very syrupy. Pour into clean, dry, warm jars and seal immediately. Take by the spoonful when required. It can also be added to hot water as a night-time toddy.

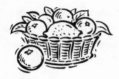

ASTHMA

There seems to be little folklore attached to such a potentially damaging affliction as asthma although there are one or two rather obscure references to sighting the devil bringing on an asthma attack. This probably related more to psychosomatic causes which had their origins in dirty deeds and a guilty conscience. Most attacks of asthma are triggered by allergic reaction, an emotional upset, anxiety or occasionally physical stress or a chesty cold.

If you have an asthma sufferer in the family you will know that there is nothing worse than that tight-chested wheeziness for which there is no magic cure but only ways of easing the discomfort, identifying the cause, reducing the risks and hoping that, as time passes, the attacks will become less frequent. The majority of asthma attacks are not serious enough to warrant admittance to hospital. However, if the patient turns blue or becomes very pale and clammy do not hesitate to dial 999. It is always better to be safe than sorry.

Cool-headed comfort is the key to reducing the misery of asthma. Do not fuss and flap and burn feathers under the victim's nose. Sit them back-to-front on an upright chair with their elbows resting on the back (this lifts the top of the rib cage, keeps it stable and allows for more efficient breathing) but do not force them to lie down. Have a couple of light cellular blankets handy which will keep the patient warm without adding suffocating weight and make sure that there is plenty of fresh air in the room. Sometimes a hot drink will work wonders. Other tried and tested nursing techniques suggest keeping the feet and hands warm, using hot water bottles or warm cloths, and asthma sufferers are helped considerably merely by the solid, comforting, quiet presence of a calm and sensible person.

Looking to the Long Term

Many of the long-term remedies given for asthma really act as cold preventatives and reduce catarrhal infection, generally improving the mind and body rather than actually curing the problem.

• *Cold water* John Wesley recommended cold baths daily and several nursing manuals suggested taking a cold bath once a fortnight but I am sure that this was put forward more in the spirit of ensuring no naughty thoughts than in improving an ailing body. Nevertheless a daily dip, preferably in the sea, does keep you fit.
• *Yoga* This brings about a state of tranquillity thus unburdening the mind of stressful thoughts.
• *Diet* Improve the diet and avoid those things which may be harmful. Chocolate, cheese, tea, coffee and cow's

milk products are thought to be detrimental although goat's milk, and yoghurt and cheese made from it, have long been considered to be of benefit to anyone suffering from chest ailments. Paradoxically, lemons are of great benefit whilst other citrus fruits may cause problems. Take additional vitamins A, E and B_6. Keep your weight down but do not diet seriously enough to create problems of anxiety or unhappiness. If there is real difficulty in preventing overweight take professional advice which will put you on the right path without causing stress.

• *Cabbages, nettles and onions* All are of benefit to the body in many ways. A good method of expressing the fresh juice from cabbage is to soak the fresh green leaf in water until well saturated then wring out the liquid and drink it daily. You will find other helpful remedies under **Catarrh**.

• *Garlic* Chew 2 garlic cloves daily though this is of less value than the following recipe.

Garlic Cure for Asthma
3 heads garlic
600ml(1 pint) water
300ml($\frac{1}{2}$ pint) cider vinegar
50g(2oz) honey or sugar

Peel the garlic cloves and simmer them gently in the water for 20 minutes. Remove, drain and place in a jar. Add the vinegar and honey or sugar to the garlicky water and boil until syrupy. Pour over the garlic in the jar and leave to cool before sealing. Take one of the cloves with the syrup each day. This remedy is also said to improve the memory.

• *Irish moss* Used in the next recipe, this is an expectorant and helps you breathe more easily.

A Honey for Breathlessness
$\frac{1}{2}$ onion
2 cloves garlic
600ml(1 pint) Irish moss jelly
$\frac{1}{2}$ cup clear honey

Peel and chop the onion and garlic then simmer gently with the Irish moss until soft. Strain and allow to cool then add $\frac{1}{2}$ cup of honey. Take daily to ensure that chestiness does not turn into asthma.

• *Liquorice root* A strong decoction of this reasonably pleasant-tasting root relieves chesty colds if drunk daily. It is certainly an improvement on the old-fashioned cure-all of $\frac{1}{2}$ pint of tar water taken daily!

• *Carrots* Whilst I think that a spartan diet of plain boiled carrots for two weeks, as advocated in days past, could be bad for you there is no doubt that a small glass of carrot juice taken daily reduces the risk of an asthma attack.

• *Castor oil cure* Whip 25g(1oz) of castor oil with 50g(2oz) of clear honey or mix 1 tablespoon of castor oil with 1 tablespoon of cider vinegar. Taken daily either remedy alleviates not only asthma symptoms but also those of catarrh and arthritis.

• *Vervain* This is the sacred flower of the Druids which magicians wear. It is believed to be able to relieve any nervous disorders, so drink a glass of vervain tea – flowers, leaf and stalk – immediately upon rising each morning.

For Immediate Relief

• *Massage* With your patient sitting back to front on the chair, as suggested earlier (page 69), massage the spine with both hands working from the bottom upwards. This relieves stress and the uncomfortable ache in back and shoulders caused by fighting for breath. Also there is a small area in the hollow of the throat which, if massaged with the little finger in a gentle circular movement without pressure, can bring almost magical relief.

• *Inhalants* The best inhalant that I know of is Friar's balsam in boiling water. Another very mild one is the leaves of mullein (*Verbascum thapsus*).

• *Teas* Thyme, marjoram, lavender, hyssop, eucalyptus, coltsfoot and lungwort are all antiseptic and break down mucus.

> *A Special Tea for Asthma*
> 1 part each cayenne, Iceland moss, thyme, red clover, liquorice and horehound
> 4 parts Irish moss

Mix together and make a tea using 1 teaspoon of the mixture to 1 cup of boiling water. Take 1 teaspoon four times daily.

• *Heart's ease, honeysuckle or lobelia* These are all old-fashioned medicines for asthma. Tinctures, teas and tablets can be bought from herbalists.

• *Old-fashioned proprietary medicines* Those which contain squills, gum ammoniacum, cayenne, capsicine (capsicum) and ipecacuanha are recommended.

• *Lemon juice* Take 1 teaspoon of hot lemon juice, with or without honey, every 15 minutes.

• *Essential oils of eucalyptus, pine, rosemary and marjoram* Blend 2 drops of each into 2 tablespoons of oil and rub into the chest. After anointing with this aromatic mixture cover with a hot, dry towel to release the full benefit and to keep the patient warm.

HAYFEVER

Hayfever sufferers need no introduction to the problem for they are only too well aware of the horrors of persistent sneezing fits, uncontrollably streaming eyes and nose, tickly cough, catarrh, headache, itchy skin and tiredness. Hayfever is caused by an allergic reaction to a substance which affects the fragile, sensitive areas of the eyes and the nose. (See **Allergic Reactions**.)

Hayfever is not a dangerous complaint. It is merely debilitating, distressing and destructive for it is virtually impossible to lead a normal life whilst suffering a prolonged bout. It also leaves a weary body vulnerable to infection and wreaks havoc upon the looks, thus leaving women particularly depressed. The best advice that can be given is to identify the provocative substance which causes the allergy as quickly as possible and keep well away from it. At one time it was thought beneficial to smoke herbal cigarettes containing stramonium which is another name for datura or thorn apple, a highly dangerous plant. Another suspect recipe which was popular and which shows the lengths to which a sufferer may be driven was that of milk, sherry and a *soupçon* of aconite (also poisonous) shaken together and sweetened to taste!

Long-term Recommendations

Most authorities would say that there is no foolproof method of guarding against allergic reaction. It would seem that commonsense dictates an improvement in one's general state of health by using better breathing techniques, improving one's posture, exercising more, giving up smoking, ensuring that one is not constipated and improving the diet in three ways. First of all spend a few days eating only citrus fruit, drinking carrot or beetroot juice and consuming lots of raw vegetables. Follow this by one week of eating no red meat, refined carbohydrate, milk products, eggs, pulses, nuts or grains. Thereafter avoid junk foods and cut down on red meats, refined carbohydrate and milk products (try soya milk instead), all of which make mucus thus exacerbating hayfever.

If you suffer from an allergy caused by natural occurrences, such as flowers in bloom or hay cutting, and know roughly the seasons in which these occur, embark on a course of honeycomb one month beforehand – 1 teaspoon chewed daily as one might chew gum for at least 15 minutes and then discarded – continuing this treatment for as long as is required. It is believed that people raised on a daily teaspoon of honeycomb will never suffer from allergy throughout their lifetime.

Garlic perles taken daily are also believed to minimize the problem as is nettle tea drunk regularly.

• *Red clover tea* Clover is recommended to control allergy therefore it might be sensible to drink this regularly when the hayfever season is approaching. Steep 1 teaspoon of fresh blossoms in 1 cup of boiling water for 10 minutes, having first made sure that any small insects have been well and truly shaken out of their habitat.

To Counter Irritation when Under Siege

Any aromatic herb or inhalant given under **Asthma** is suitable.

• *Lemon juice* Sea water sniffed up each nostril daily is said to minimize allergy but sniffing lemon juice up each nostril at the onset of an attack, as advocated by some, is a mind-bending experience. I can only say that such was my state of mind when I tried this remedy that I believe I stopped sneezing and went into shock. It is kinder and more practical to plug each nostril with cotton wool soaked in lemon juice which also reduces the chances of catching a cold. Sniffing snuff was once used to counteract the sneezes by producing a whole range of self-inflicted ones.

• *Aromatic inhalant* A mixture of 25g(1oz) each of eucalyptus leaves, marsh mallow flowers and sweet violets, boiled in 600ml(1 pint) of water and inhaled beneath a towel is a refreshingly pleasant experience.

• *Pine and eucalyptus* Infuse a pinch each of pine and eucalyptus leaves, in 600ml(1 pint) of boiling water and take during an attack.

• *Elecampane tea* Elecampane is a robust, golden, daisy-type plant which is still used in many proprietary cough medicines. Use 25g(1oz) to 600ml(1 pint) of boiling water to make a soothing tea which should be drunk at the rate of ½ wineglass every four hours or used as a vapour inhalant.

• *Rose hips* These are full of valuable vitamin C to replace that used up during a hayfever attack.

• *Rose hip tea* For an overwhelmingly

delicious and colourful tea take 2 tablespoons of commercially prepared dried rosehips, place them in a small china bowl and cover with water. Leave for 12 hours. Bring 1.8 litres(3 pints) of water to the boil in a stainless steel or enamel pan, add the rose hips and 2 teaspoons of hibiscus flowers (which add glorious colour and a lemony tang) and simmer gently for half an hour. Strain and keep in a china tea pot in the refrigerator. Reheat when needed but keep no longer than three days.

Rose Hip Syrup
450g(1lb) bright orange hips picked just after the second frost
boiling water
honey

Crush the hips and put them into 900ml(1½ pints) of boiling water (do not use an iron or aluminium pan: one should never cook with aluminium and especially not if one suffers from asthma). Bring to the boil then stand off the heat for 15 minutes. Strain through several layers of muslin, reserving the juice. Reboil the mashed fruit again with a further 300ml(½ pint) of water. Stand for a further 15 minutes and strain. Mix the two juices together, return to the pan and reduce by a long slow boiling until there is approximately 600ml(1 pint) of syrup left. Sweeten to taste with honey and bottle in clean dry containers. Keep refrigerated once open.

● *Goose grease and golden rod* This lotion was used to soothe noses and lips made sore by constant sneezing and wiping. It was also believed to trap offending pollen and protect the sensitive area. The herbal moisturizer recommended under **Allergic Reactions** is also very effective.

● *Olive oil* A gentle salve based on this oil will soothe inflamed eyelids. Occasionally irritation and inflammation of the eyes can be caused by conjunctivitis which may also be the result of an allergic reaction.

Eye Salve
50g(2oz) white wax (paraffin wax or beeswax)
300ml(½ pint) virgin olive oil
100ml(2 fl oz) pure white vinegar

Melt the wax and oil together in one small bowl over boiling water and in another gently warm the vinegar in the same way. Remove both bowls from the heat and beat the vinegar slowly into the oily mixture. Continue to beat gently until cool. Transfer to a pot and seal when cold.

ECZEMA

Eczema is most usually caused by an allergic reaction to any one of the substances referred to under **Allergic Reactions**. Man-made fibres, cheap jewellery, metal zippers, nickel, zinc, aluminium, lanolin and specific plants such as poison ivy, hellebore, hog weed and primrose are particularly likely to bring on this condition which can vary from a mild red irritation to small but extremely unpleasant blisters which join up to form large weeping patches which then crust over and flake again. Olden-day psychologists believed that the area of the eruption was pre-ordained by inner problems: on the face

73

betokened overweening vanity, around the mouth meant that you had been speaking ill of someone, itchy feet showed a desire to run away, on the hands meant overwork and anxiety, whilst on the neck it denoted a longing for pretty things. This diagnosis was not too difficult to work out really, and such were the yardsticks by which witches were hounded to death. Nevertheless, eczema is considered to be the outer manifestation of emotional and physical problems not yet come to light. Diet should be examined and refined as for asthma and hayfever and highly spiced food, pickles and alcohol should be avoided. Constipation and problems with the kidneys are also thought to be contributory factors in eczema.

Children, particularly bottle-fed babies, occasionally suffer from a milk allergy which causes eczema. Some authorities suggest that ½ a teaspoon of sunflower oil a day will cure the problem and are adamant that cow's milk is the cause. Others suggest rubbing a little oil of evening primrose into the affected area to help it heal quickly. If eczema is diagnosed, safe infusions suitable for a baby's bath water are marigold and camomile. Use a few drops of a prepared tincture or an essential oil. If the condition persists consult your health visitor again.

Old-fashioned remedies, of which there are many, vary from the moderate starch poultice or strips of linen soaked in olive oil to reduce scabbing, to starch and talcum powder or tar ointment in vaseline to dress and soothe. The less humane remedies included strapping children's arms to their sides so that they could not scratch! Two eminently sensible and safe ideas are to wash in water and oatmeal (which cleanses without irritation) and to dress the itchy areas with calamine lotion.

Two-Way Remedies

● *Marigold, sage or camomile* These three healing herbs can either be drunk several times a day to soothe the beleaguered spirit or used as an infusion to bathe the irritated area. Essential oil of camomile diluted in almond oil may be rubbed into the skin to promote healing.
● *Cabbage* The juice may be drunk daily or take the well-pulped leaves of a fresh, green Savoy.
● *Carrots* Eaten raw in salads they will do much to promote a healthy body, as will the juice. A poultice made of raw grated carrots is a very old remedy for skin complaints which even today is still used in some beauty parlours.
● *Bilberries* Settlers travelling to new countries made sure that they took a good supply of bilberries with them for they were an indispensable part of country medicine. Drink the juice or chew a few dried berries at a time to clear the skin of blemishes. Or make the following strong decoction to drink in the quantities of 1 small glass hourly. Place 50g(2oz) of dried bilberries in a stainless steel pan with 900ml(1½ pints) of lukewarm water and leave to stand for 1 hour. Bring slowly to the boil and boil for 20 minutes then remove from the heat and leave until soft. Strain and use as needed. It may also be used as a healing skin cleanser.
● *Slippery elm* Slippery elm soap was used to replace soaps which contained damaging animal fats and chemicals. A little of the powdered bark mixed with warm water will give a healing paste which can be used on the hands and other sore places at night, whilst an emollient glass of slippery elm and honey taken each morning before breakfast may prove to be a necessary

laxative: 1 dessertspoon of each, whisked into hot water and seasoned with a pinch of cayenne. Both English elm (*Ulmus campestris*) and American elm (*Ulmus fulva*) are almost endangered species since the plague of Dutch elm disease and are, thankfully, being left at present to regenerate.

● *Birch leaves* Simmer 50g(2oz) of birch leaves in 1 litre(1¾ pints) of water for three minutes. Leave until hand hot then add a pinch of bicarbonate of soda. Allow to cool for several hours before using as a useful disinfectant wash and a therapeutic daily drink.

● *Watercress* Eat regularly and use the juice to wash the affected areas. The juice can be either expressed fresh or extracted by placing in cold water, bringing to the boil and gently simmering for 10 minutes. Leave to cool.

Remedies to Take

Try the famous 'green cocktail' (see under **Body Odour**) but include also some beetroot and parsley.

● *Nettle or dandelion* Drink the tea of either plant. Alternatively eat the nettles in a nourishing soup, and chop the well-washed dandelion leaves into a salad of cucumber and watercress, which are also expressly recommended to alleviate eczema.

● *Horehound* For many years the chopped leaves of horehound were added to the diet in order to clear the blood of impurities when a skin disease was in evidence. However, as the generic term *Murrubium* from the Hebrew word for 'bitter' makes clear, the leaves taste unpleasant as well as being hairy. Horehound tea well sweetened with honey is a better idea.

● *Goat's milk* This can be a valuable addition to the diet for anyone suffering from an allergy.

● *Evening primrose oil* Amongst many other things this remarkable cure-all reduces tension and stress.

● *Burdock* An infusion of burdock can be used to bathe damaged skin and burdock and camomile drink (see page 167) will strengthen the body against skin irritations if a small cup is drunk four times a day for two weeks.

● *Daisy infusion* Place 25g(1oz) of daisies in 1 litre(1¾ pints) of water and bring gently to the boil. Boil for two minutes. Remove from the heat and leave to infuse for 10 minutes. Drink 3 cups a day between meals. Could this be the same daisy wine once recommended for concussion (see page 40)?

● *Red clover and heart's ease* Use the two together, with or without marigold, to make a gentle infusion for alleviating stress.

Soothing Lotions and Potions

● *Walnut leaves* Use an infusion of 15g(½oz) of fresh leaves to 600ml(1 pint) water to bathe the affected area daily.

● *Speedwell* An infusion of 1 teaspoon of the dried herb to 1 cup of water can be used to bathe the afflicted part morning and night.

● *Flax (linseed)* Add it to the bath water to soften the skin and act as a tranquillizer. Boil 50g(2oz) of linseed in 1 litre(1¾ pints) of water for just two minutes. Strain and use the liquid.

● *Essential oil of rose* Added to the bath water this has the same effect as flax (above) with the extra attraction of a delightful fragrance.

● *Wheatgerm and vitamin E oils* These are now used extensively to heal damaged skin.

Allergies

- *Milk whey* This will reduce irritation when used to clean dry skin.
- *Lavender oil* Fill a glass jar ¾ full of lavender flowers and pour in enough virgin olive oil to practically fill the jar. Put in a double boiler and heat gently for two hours. Cool in the pan then filter. Store in small bottles in a dark place and use regularly on sore spots.

Body Odour and Bad Breath

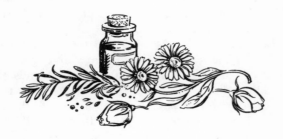

Body Odour

Old folk remedies for body odour are scarce not because of modesty but rather because it was an accepted fact of life. Few washing facilities existed either for body or clothes and the atmosphere was heavy with the smells of open fires and cooking. Even the highly born, except for an enlightened few, viewed placing water on the skin with a certain amount of trepidation. However, in today's society cleanliness is next to godliness and with the marvels of modern plumbing in most homes and a battery of anti-perspirants and deodorants to choose from there is little excuse to be otherwise. My own opinion is that soap and water daily is essential and that there is nothing worse than a highly perfumed deodorant overlaying the smell of sweat. Many people do not need to use either anti-perspirants or deodorants and an increasing number are finding that they are becoming resistant or developing allergies to them. Synthetic fabrics and tight-fitting clothes increase the likelihood of excess perspiration and body odour, and an overindulgence in highly spiced and flavoured foods can create a transitory but noticeable odour exuded through the pores. Eating plenty of raw, dark green, leafy vegetables, including parsley, will reduce body odours caused by eating curry, garlic and onions, or try the famous 'green cocktail' described below.

Intake to Reduce Output

- *Green cocktail* Place a good selection of green vegetables into a blender with the addition of carrots, peppers, tomatoes, plenty of seasoning, the juice of 1 lemon and a little water. Blend well and dilute if necessary. These leafy green vegetables not only contain a lot of chlorophyll which will dispel bad odours but they also have a laxative and diuretic effect, thus purifying the whole system.

● *Fenugreek tea* Two level teaspoons of fenugreek seeds to one cup of boiling water, allowed to infuse for five minutes then stirred and strained into another cup and taken daily, with or without honey, is what Middle Eastern ladies drink to make themselves desirable. It helps to purify the blood, reduces bad breath and body odour and significantly improves catarrhal and sinus conditions. If used daily the fragrant, slightly spicy, smell of fenugreek will eventually permeate the skin.

● *Lovage tea, chrysanthemum tea or sage tea* These are all excellent remedies to reduce body odour as are many of the teas suggested for anxiety – one of the reasons that we 'break out in a sweat'.

A Tonic to Purify
the System and Reduce
Bad Breath and Body Odour
1 tablespoon crushed blueberries
1 tablespoon shredded watercress
1 tablespoon sassafras bark
300ml($\frac{1}{2}$ pint) boiling water

Pour the boiling water over the other ingredients. Cover, leave to cool then strain. Take 1 cup four times a day for one day and during this 24 hour period eat only very light meals and drink only mineral water.

● *Nettles* Nettle beer is a gypsy remedy. A small glass taken daily keeps the body fit and healthy and is also the reason why most old-fashioned country folk, contrary to popular obloquy, smelt so clean.

Nettle Beer
900g(2lb) young nettles
2 lemons
4.75 litres(8 pints) water
450g(1lb) demerara sugar
25g(1oz) cream of tartar
brewer's yeast prepared in advance according to manufacturer's instructions
a plastic bucket with a lid

Use the tops of the nettles only. Put them into a large enamel saucepan with the thinly pared rinds of the lemons – use a potato peeler for this job. Add the water and bring to the boil. Boil for 20 minutes then strain the liquid through a nylon sieve on to the sugar and the cream of tartar in a plastic bucket with a lid. Stir well and when lukewarm add the lemon juice and prepared yeast. Cover and leave in a warm room for three days then transfer to a cooler place for two days. Syphon into strong bottles – large glass beer or cider bottles are best but do not use plastic soft drink bottles for they will not sustain the pressure. If the beer ferments vigorously keep the tops, either screw or cork, loose for a day or two before sealing down. Keep in a cool, outside place (garage or outhouse) for a week before drinking.

Natural Deodorants

● *Cleavers (or goosegrass)* This is the most old-fashioned natural deodorant and one of the few, with its sister plants of lady's bedstraw and sweet woodruff, mentioned in ancient herbals as being suitable for keeping house, clothes and body sweet smelling – cleavers for washing, lady's bedstraw for strewing and stuffing in mattresses and sweet woodruff for placing in linen cupboards and drawers.

• *A natural deodorant* Take a large handful of cleavers and put it into a pan with 1 litre(1¾ pints) of water. Bring gently to the boil and simmer for 15 minutes. Leave to get cold then strain. It will keep for at least a week in the refrigerator but the plant is so common it can be made right through the summer. Apply with cotton wool or a spray.

Lavender Deodorant
3 drops essential oil of lavender
1 tablespoon sugar
600ml(1 pint) distilled or cold boiled water

Put all together in a bottle, seal, shake well and leave for two weeks. Always shake well before using either on cotton wool or in a spray.

• *Witch hazel* Use it neat provided it does not irritate the skin and dilute with water for a useful antiseptic underarm aftershave.
• *Thyme, rosemary, eau de Cologne mint or lavender* Take a large handful of any one of these sweet-smelling, antiseptic herbs and place in a pan with enough water to cover. Simmer for 5 minutes, pour into a jug and stand until cold. Strain and bottle.
• *Apple cider vinegar* Mix together equal quantities of vinegar and water. Apply on cotton wool and leave for a few minutes to allow the smell to dissipate.
• *Powdered alum* A cheap and effective old-fashioned deodorant can be made from ½ teaspoon of powdered alum and 300ml(½ pint) of warm water.
• *Essential oils of thyme, marjoram, geranium, verbena, lavender, sandalwood, angelica, cinnamon and cassia* A few drops of any one of these antiseptic oils in the warm bath water will reduce

body odour and individually they have other delightful effects.
• *Cleansing bath bag* Take 3 handfuls each of dandelion leaves and stinging nettles, 2 handfuls each of blackcurrant leaves and scented geraniums. Tie into a muslin drawstring bath bag (a large white cotton handkerchief will do) and leave under the bath water as it runs. Fresh lovage or any other deliciously fragrant, antiseptic herbs can be used in the same way.

Seaweed Gel
1.25 litres(2½ pints) fresh Irish moss or carragheen
1.5 litres(3 pints) water
2 tablespoons scented floral or herb water

Soak the seaweed in fresh water and wash it well. Put it into a large pan with the measured water and bring gently to the boil. Cover and simmer for 30 minutes. Rub the gelatinous result through a fine sieve and stir in the scented water. Pour into jars when cold and keep refrigerated. This is a deodorizing gel which should be rubbed all over the body instead of soap, then rinsed off in shower or bath. It is also excellent for relieving aches and pains.

SMELLY FEET

Those of us who have seen a room cleared by the removal of a pair of shoes will know that there is no other way to describe what for some people is an unfortunate physical condition and for which they should seek professional advice. The prime offenders are lazy adolescent boys and the main cause is synthetic socks and shoes. Anyone who has spent hours tracking down an unpleasant smell in the house and

Body Odour and Bad Breath

found the culprits to be a pair of sweat-soaked nylon socks stuffed into a pair of soggy trainers will know exactly what I mean. Not only is this antisocial, but sweating feet habitually encased in synthetics can lead to athlete's foot. Whenever possible insist upon socks which contain a high percentage of cotton and try when finance and fashion allow to buy leather or canvas shoes.

Fresh Answers

- *Essential oil of lavender or lemon grass* A few drops of either in a footbath of warm water is antiseptic and deodorizing. An excellent therapy before a party is to massage the feet with a few drops of either of these oils, diluted in a little sunflower oil.
- *White willow bark* Use an infusion of this herb with a pinch of borax added as a footbath.
- *Powdered alum* Half a teaspoon to 300ml(½ pint) of warm water effectively reduces sweating and deodorizes. Dust the feet with alum powder to ensure immunity for some time.
- *Foot massage* Massage clean feet with a mixture of 6 tablespoons of witch hazel and 1 tablespoon each of tincture of arnica and glycerine. Do not use on broken skin.

BAD BREATH

In bygone days, as a result of bad teeth, disease, unhealthy food and none of the accoutrements of oral hygiene, a very great percentage of the population suffered from bad breath (halitosis) and attempted to counteract the problem with a variety of breath fresheners ranging from sweet pellets of cloves and myrrh to cachous of rose and violet. The latter of course created a sickly odour which did nothing to remove the underlying causes of which halitosis is the result.

Eating strongly flavoured foods such as garlic, onion, cheese and beer leaves an immediate smell on the breath which is reasonably transitory but bad breath caused by smoking, catarrh, sinus infection, tooth decay, tonsillitis, constipation and stomach disorders requires a cleansing and a clearing to get the body working properly. As any Victorian nanny would unequivocally have stated, 'clean breath and a clear mind are the signs of a healthy body'.

Instant Answers

If the problem is digestive or a temporarily upset stomach then ½ teaspoon of kaolin powder or a few drops of essential oil of peppermint in a glass of warm water will soothe and improve matters.

If the cause of halitosis is a sore throat either honey and lemon or a few drops of oil of cloves in hot water, to first gargle with and then swallow, will kill bacteria.

Any of the following chewed well will disguise the smell of recently eaten foods: parsley, mint, cardamom, cloves, aniseed, juniper berries, an apple, coffee beans, fennel seeds. All of these can also have the long-term effect of improving tummy upsets.

Morning-After Remedies

- *Yoghurt* A large tablespoon of plain live yoghurt works wonders. A bowl of it will also cure the most devastating hangovers.
- *Coffee* Grind the fresh beans with a few cardamom seeds and make into a reviving cup to be drunk without milk

80

first thing in the morning (but avoid if you also have a hangover).

Breath Freshener
150ml(¼ pint) sherry
15g(½oz) each ground cloves and nutmeg
pinch each ground cinnamon and caraway

Seal tightly together in a bottle and shake frequently for one week. This tincture should be taken, a few drops at a time, on a sugar lump or in hot water to sweeten the most dire morning-after breath.

Mouthwashes

● *Hydrogen peroxide* One teaspoon added to a glass of warm water, with or without 1 teaspoon of sea salt, is a very cleansing gargle and mouthwash. Avoid swallowing.
● *Bicarbonate of soda and sea salt* One teaspoon of each in a glass of warm water makes an effective mouthwash.
● *Cider vinegar, tincture of myrrh and oil of cloves* A quarter of a cup of cider vinegar, 1 tablespoon of clear honey and 3 drops each of tincture of myrrh and oil of cloves, diluted with a little hot water, makes an antiseptic mouthwash and gargle which can be safely swallowed.
● *Eucalyptus oil, oil of cloves and tincture of myrrh* Six drops of oil of eucalyptus

and 2 drops each oil of cloves and tincture of myrrh shaken together with 600ml(1 pint) of hot water then bottled and kept handy in the bathroom is very refreshing first thing in the morning.
● *Lavender, marjoram, summer savoury, thyme and rosemary* Separately or combined in a vinegar or infusion these antiseptic and sweet-smelling herbs are safe and pleasant to use.

Long-Term Solutions

Do not drink water with meals as this upsets the gastric juices.

Exercise, fresh air and deep breathing stimulate a good supply of oxygen to the system.

Visit the dentist regularly.

Examine yourself for stress problems or a poor digestive reaction to certain foods.

● *Syrup of figs* One teaspoon in hot water each night until the breath is sweet has much the same effect as sweet liquorice water from the Middle East.
● *Lemon pips* An old-fashioned remedy to kill worms (which cause notoriously bad breath) in small children was to simmer these in honey and spoon down the gooey mixture whilst still warm.
● *Quince seeds* Simmer the seeds in water until soft. Strain, gargle with and swallow the liquid.

Problems of Digestion

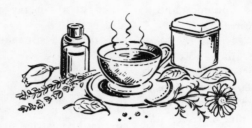

Indigestion

Over the years whilst compiling information for this book I have realized that there are many differing views on what constitutes a particular ailment, and never has it been more apparent than in the search for potions to remedy indigestion. To further complicate matters there are other variables to be taken into consideration: the state of mind of the sufferer, the variety of foodstuffs which exacerbate individual digestive problems and a complexity of aches and pains which are frequently held to be responsible for or to be a direct result of indigestion. I shall therefore do as many old wives and modern doctors have done and put acidity, dyspepsia, flatulence, heartburn, colicky pains and general excessive windiness all under the heading of **Indigestion**.

The symptoms can vary from pains in the chest to a distended midriff, from a hearty belch to ominous internal rumblings, from stomach ache and nausea to that unbearable burning surge of acidity into the mouth and the general feeling of malaise that makes you wish that you had eaten and drunk perhaps a little less well and a little more wisely.

There is no doubt however that several specific circumstances can cause indigestion. Eating when you are in a state of tension, taking food 'on the run', getting up and down from a meal, swallowing food too quickly without chewing it thoroughly, taking water with meals which upsets the gastric juices and sitting badly or eating food on a tray on your lap whilst hunched over the television set, which causes the intestine to become squashed, are all prime causes of the above agonies. Eating late at night can lead to a bad case of night-time heebie jeebies when the pain is so bad that some sufferers have believed themselves to be in the throes of a heart attack. Women are more prone to indigestion during the time of their periods whilst sufferers from chronic constipation also feel the pangs rather more frequently than do other folk. Smoking can also be considered a contributory factor especially when it is allied to an empty stomach, black coffee and stress at work.

If you find the cause for your problem amongst the above suggestions then self-help is entirely in your hands but there may be other causes which are purely dietary. An immoderate consumption of rich food and alcohol may seem worth the risk at the time but be sure that you have an antidote to hand. If however the problem persists beyond the normal time expected to overcome such indulgence examine your diet for specifics: fatty foods, red meat, pork, coffee, tea, red wine, sherry, smoked and very salty foods, acidic fruit (oranges, tomatoes) and commercially produced foods which contain a high percentage of food additives. Gin taken with tonic water has also been known to have an unholy effect on the digestion as do many wines and beers which contain chemicals.

To some extent we have brought these problems upon ourselves by relegating many of the old-fashioned herb and spice combinations that accompanied our meals to the realms of fuddy-duddy tradition. Roast pork for instance was cooked with sage and onion not only to lend it flavour but also to provide a very necessary insurance against indigestion when one was eating a rich meat. In France it is almost traditional to follow roast pork with an open apple tart and a glass of calvados and in northern European countries both pork and certain dense cheeses are prepared with caraway to give a distinctive flavour and to aid digestion. Two other favourites are pork or ham seasoned with juniper, and sauerkraut served with pork. Both the Germans and the Japanese have learned the benefits to the digestive system of fermented cabbage (although I personally have my own views on the matter).

Greens, particularly the strong dark varieties, were the vegetables most frequently served with Sunday lunch and the water in which they were cooked was used to make the gravy which accompanied the meat, and this same liquid can be drunk as an antidote to heartburn.

A traditional accompaniment to roast beef is mustard which will help a heavy meat be more easily digested. Both horseradish and freshly ground black pepper have much the same effect and if you are in the habit of eating cold roast beef sandwiches it is essential that you add one of this trio.

Sage leaves are traditionally used when cooking liver and kidneys as it fixes their high iron content and makes them more digestible. Both types of offal should be left to soak well in cold water for at least two hours before cooking. I had always thought that when my mother added a tablespoon of vinegar to the water this was done to tenderize the offal but I now realize that it was probably the tail end of a long-held belief that as liver and kidneys are eliminative organs the vinegar would rid them of their toxins.

Parsley, sage, thyme, garlic, marjoram, onions and lemon were and still should be used to stuff poultry and game, particularly if you have a good healthy free-range bird, for they all help to cut the richness and help digestion in the same way as the astringent cranberry and redcurrant do for turkey and game. Rich oily fish baked with fennel, creamy sauces seasoned with dill and many other gourmet dishes had their beginnings in practicalities rather than in haute cuisine. Although many spices and herbs were used to disguise the taste of stale meat and to counteract its effect upon the consumer, those warm Oriental spices such as cumin, coriander, cinnamon, fenugreek and cayenne were also used to add piquancy to the palate and power to the digestion when a long feast was in progress.

Many people are allergic to certain foods and drinks but getting the 'burps' when we have eaten cucumber is usually as a result of having peeled it, for the skin normally acts as its own built-in digestive. In fact we should not peel many of the fruits and vegetables we eat. Apples and carrots are both valuable additions to the diet and also keep our bodies working smoothly but they are more effective if they are left unpeeled – although with today's proliferation of pesticides it is necessary to make sure that they are well scrubbed in several changes of water.

Raw grated carrot is considered a trustworthy antidote to dyspepsia and so are fennel and parsley although I am certain that the notorious radish and spring onion could do battle with the most iron constitution and win. Both celery and fresh pineapple, eaten at the end of a meal, will improve the digestive processes.

For some unhappy sufferers from indigestion the cause may be far more difficult to identify. Although we usually know what we are allergic to, some conditions can be created by the wrong combination of foods eaten at the same time. One of the most potentially damaging meals can be steak with baked potato or chips and salad, followed by a sweet fruit dessert. A steak eaten with a bread roll can, I am assured, take up to 90 hours to be digested and eventually eliminated from the body. This is because the digestive juices can't easily cope with this combination of foods. Some people cannot tolerate cheese and

fruit together whilst others baulk at a meat sandwich with pickles. Unrefined carbohydrates and whole milk may also create problems. Bread made with quick-rise yeast can also upset the digestion quite considerably.

Although alcohol – particularly some of the nasty chemical varieties on the market – will not do you a lot of good when taken in excess an aperitif taken before a meal, a glass of good white wine with the meal and a digestif to follow were and still are considered to be not only a civilized pleasure but an exquisite necessity for the well-being of the body. Unfortunately, as is the case with so many good things, we cannot resist an occasional overindulgence.

If you suffer from indigestion which is persistent or if it should become progressively worse you should take professional advice.

Aid and Antidote

Eat plenty of raw grated carrots, fennel, parsley and green vegetables if you suffer from dyspepsia. The water in which well-washed new potatoes have been cooked or the cooking-water from dark green turnip tops will counteract acidity.

If you like wholemeal bread but it does not like you try adding well-crushed coriander, caraway, aniseed or fennel seeds to the basic dough.

Chew black peppercorns or suck liquorice wood slowly.

● *Apple cider vinegar or lemon juice* One teaspoon of either in ½ cup of warm water every 15 minutes will relieve acidity and heartburn. This may seem to be fighting fire with fire but using antacids provokes the body into producing yet more acid.
● *Bicarbonate of soda* One teaspoon in

hot water relieves heartburn, acidity and dyspepsia. An even better method is to mix 2 tablespoons of bicarbonate of soda with 1 teaspoon of ground ginger and take 1 teaspoon of this mixture in hot water before breakfast.

● *Carbonated lemonade* The old-fashioned colourless variety drunk warm relieves flatulence and stomach ache.

● *Soda water* This relieves flatulence and the type of fuzzy headache that sometimes goes with indigestion.

● *Water* Drinking lots of water dispels heartburn. Lemon barley water and pure lemonade taken by the small glassful will also help.

● *Barley water, oats or porridge* All of these will settle flatulence and heartburn.

● *Yoghurt* The plain live variety will soothe digestive disorders.

● *Goat's milk* This will ease persistent heartburn and flatulence.

● *Slippery elm* To soothe and reduce acidity mix 1 teaspoon of the powdered bark to a paste with a little cold water and add to 1 cup of boiling water. Season with nutmeg or cinnamon to taste and sweeten with honey.

● *Charcoal* Charcoal biscuits or tablets are a very old-fashioned remedy for wind, heartburn and more severe tummy troubles, especially nausea. Powdered chalk was also used as an antidote for acidity and although I cannot recommend the latter both the charcoal biscuits and the tablets are easily available and are invaluable.

● *Cloves* A drop or two of oil of cloves in hot water, 6 cloves steeped in a cup of boiling water and drunk as a tea or the cloves chewed as they are will all dispel pain and flatulence. They will also make the breath smell sweeter.

● *Ginger* Soak 1 teaspoon of freshly grated ginger in a cup of boiling water. Stand for 10 minutes and drink warm.

● *Fenugreek tea* This tea is specially good if a catarrhal condition is the cause of digestive problems.

● *Garlic* One clove of garlic should be crushed or chopped into 300ml($\frac{1}{2}$ pint) of boiling water. Cooking with garlic will also reduce the chances of digestive problems and I suspect that this very useful remedy may also have been used as an antidote to food poisoning.

● *Bay tea* Take 2 bay leaves and the peel of $\frac{1}{2}$ a well-washed orange, cover with 150ml($\frac{1}{4}$ pint) of boiling water and leave to stand for 10 minutes. Strain and drink warm. If you are prone to digestive problems use bay leaves in cooking as much as possible.

● *Angelica* Sweet, musky angelica was considered to be a forceful weapon against the plague. The fresh stem can be chewed raw to alleviate stomach pains but make sure that it is angelica from your garden and not its lookalike hemlock gathered in the wild which would assure the contrary result. Avoid taking angelica just before retiring as it is also a stimulant and may keep you awake.

● *Cardamom* To dispel flatulence chew the seeds as they are or simmer 6 pods with a pinch of ground ginger or grated nutmeg in 2 cups of water. Cardamom seeds crushed and kept in with the fresh coffee will also reduce the chances of indigestion.

● *Camomile tea* A tea which calms and soothes. Add a pinch of allspice and 1 teaspoon of honey for extra benefit, especially for children.

● *Cinnamon* Half a teaspoon of ground cinnamon in 1 cup of warm milk with honey or cinnamon tea made with hot water will dispel windiness in all degrees.

● *Caraway* Crush 1oz(25g) of caraway seeds and leave them to steep overnight in 600ml(1 pint) of boiling water.

Strain, bottle and keep refrigerated to relieve the misery of wind and heartburn.

• *Peppermint* A few drops of oil of peppermint in hot water will relieve pain and flatulence. Peppermint tea made with 1 teaspoon of the herb to 1 cup of boiling water will also bring relief. Peppermint also relieves period pains.

• *Marjoram* If you suffer from digestive disorders always cook your meat with marjoram when appropriate or make a tea with 1 teaspoon of the fresh leaves to 1 cup of boiling water. All varieties of marjoram are extremely easy to grow in the garden and make superb variegated rockery plants which the bees love. Thyme should also be used in exactly the same way but for other meats, especially game and poultry.

• *Basil* Use basil in cooking and particularly chopped on tomato salads to reduce the risk of acid heartburn. Make a basil tea with 1 teaspoon of the fresh herb to 1 cup of boiling water or even more deliciously macerate 1 handful of fresh basil in 1 litre(1¾ pints) of white wine for three days. Strain and rebottle and take one small glassful after meals.

• *Hop syrup* Many people suffer from acidity, heartburn and dyspepsia after drinking beer and lager, especially those containing a high percentage of chemicals. Perhaps the following old-fashioned remedy is the answer. Brew 1 cup of strong hop tea with 1 tablespoon of glycerine. Stir well, cover and steep for five minutes. Strain and drink one hour before meals.

• *Mustard* Amongst country folk one of the prime remedies for a painful digestive problem was to nibble the leaf of wild mustard which was searingly fiery enough for the remedy to have stated that good draughts of water be taken withal. We now know that we should eat mustard with food that may be difficult to digest but a tea made with mustard seed is also remarkably beneficial. To 1 cup of hop tea add 1 teaspoon of mustard seeds. Leave to steep and drink warm with the seed which should be swallowed. Take ½ cup twice a day before meals.

• *Aniseed* Make some aniseed tea in the proportions of 1 teaspoon of the crushed seeds to 1 cup of boiling water. Or make a syrup by boiling 2 tablespoons of crushed aniseed and 2 tablespoons of honey in 600ml(1 pint) of water. Take 2 tablespoons of the tea or syrup before each meal. Both of these relieve heartburn and flatulence.

• *Juniper* The berries steeped in hot water or 1 tablespoon of gin taken in hot water will bring relief from stomach ache and flatulence.

Juniper Syrup
100g(4oz) juniper berries
a piece of finely pared lemon rind
1 litre(1¾ pints) water
2 tablespoons honey

Simmer the berries and peel in the water until they are soft. Press as much of the mixture as is possible without undue force through a fine sieve. Stir in the honey and reheat the mixture to boiling point. Store in a sealed jar in the refrigerator and take 1 tablespoon after meals.

• *Sage* Use this herb when cooking fatty meats and offal or make a tea with the leaves.

Sage Tonic for Wind and Fevers
25g(1oz) torn sage leaves
50g(2oz) clear honey
3 tablespoons fresh lemon juice
1 litre(1¾ pints) boiling water

Put all the ingredients into a jug, cover and leave to stand for one hour. Strain and keep refrigerated. Use hot or cold and take by the teaspoon as often as needed.

Sage and Cider Jelly
50g(2oz) dried sage
150ml(¼ pint) boiling water
450ml(¾ pint) sweet cider
900g(2lb) unrefined cane sugar
150ml(¼ pint) liquid pectin
a few pieces of fresh sage

Crumble the dried sage, put it into a china bowl and cover with the boiling water. Leave to stand for 15 minutes then strain through a muslin cloth. Put into a large saucepan and add the cider and sugar. Heat gently and stir well until the sugar has dissolved then bring to the boil. Pour in the pectin, stirring constantly, and take care that the whole lot does not boil over. Boil hard for one minute and remove from the heat. Skim and leave to stand for several minutes. Half fill hot, dry, *sterile* jars with the cooling liquid. Pop a decoratively shaped and clean piece of sage into each jar and fill up. Seal when cold. This jelly has a delicious and unique flavour but more to the point it improves the digestibility of cold pork, goose and ham.

● *Coriander* One teaspoon of the crushed seeds in 1 cup of boiling water will relieve indigestion. So will the leaves if scattered in a salad.
● *Fennel and dill* Both of these herbs are constituents of gripe water for babies. Take a large dose in hot water to get rid of windiness and hiccoughs. A tea made from 1 teaspoon of either fresh herb to 1 cup of boiling water will also help.

An Elixir to Relieve Flatulence
15g(½oz) fennel seeds
15g(½oz) coriander seeds
15g(½oz) aniseed
15g(½oz) caraway seeds
15g(½oz) angelica seeds
1 litre(1¾ pints) brandy or *eau de vie*

Make sure that the dried seeds are freshly bought from a good source: stale herbs will turn the mixture musty. Put all the ingredients in a large jar, seal and leave to macerate for two weeks. Filter and take by the small glassful when necessary. This recipe is also reputed to increase the flow of milk to nursing mothers!

● *Mint* Mint tea made in the proportions of 1 teaspoon of fresh mint to 1 cup of boiling water with a pinch of powdered ginger added is very comforting in a crisis. Cold mint tea without the ginger is a most refreshing drink in the summer and mint sauce is a very necessary accompaniment to lamb, particularly shoulder of lamb and lamb chops which can be extremely fatty.
● *Gilly flower syrup* This syrup is recommended to cure stomach pains and wind. The recipe can be found on page 59.

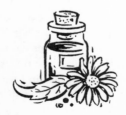

A Syrup for the Gripes
1 cup each of raisins and prunes
2 litres(3¼ pints) water
1 cup red grape juice
2 peeled sliced lemons
honey

Leave the fruit to stand in the water overnight. Pour the fruit and water into a pan with the grape juice and lemon slices and simmer until very soft. Pass through a sieve, return to the pan with enough honey to sweeten and bring to the boil. Pour into warm jars then seal when cold and keep refrigerated. Take a spoonful when necessary. It probably relieves constipation as much as indigestion.

Cranberry and Crab Apple Jelly with Thyme
500g(1lb 2oz) cranberries
500g(1lb 2oz) crab apples
1 large bunch fresh thyme
2 large lemons
water
cane sugar

Wash the cranberries and wash and slice the apples. Take two thirds of the thyme and crush it well to release the pungent oils. Squeeze the juice from the lemons and reserve. Put the pips into a preserving pan (not aluminium) with both fruits, the thyme and just enough water to cover. Simmer gently until all the fruit is very soft (it may require 'mashing' to assist it and you may need to add a little more water). Turn into a jelly bag and leave to drain overnight into a clean china bowl. The next day measure the juice and for every 600ml(1 pint) of liquid take 450g(1lb) of warmed sugar and 2 tablespoons of the lemon juice. Return all the juices to the pan and heat gently, adding the sugar and stirring well until it is dissolved. Bring to the boil and boil hard until a set is obtained. Skim and half fill hot, dry, sterilized jars with the jelly adding a decorative sprig of the remaining thyme to each jar. Wait until it begins to jell then fill up with the remainder of the jelly. Seal when cold. This is an excellent, piquant jelly to eat with rich game meats and turkey, both hot and cold. It assists in the digestion of those creatures which have been hung and cooked in rich sauces.

HICCOUGHS

Hiccoughs or hiccups can be a source of merriment, embarrassment and intense irritation and they can if they last for too long become exhausting and painful. They are caused by a nervous spasmodic contraction of the diaphragm which causes the victim to inhale suddenly and the vocal cords to close quickly, thus creating the 'hic' which is followed by the relaxation of the muscles and the 'cough'. Most attacks of hiccoughs are only of short duration although in some cases have been known to become almost permanent.

The cures for hiccoughs are legion and many of them almost come into the category of party games. I know of only two that work very well, one of which has a perfect physical explanation while the other I believe is psychological.

When an attack of hiccoughs starts take a paper bag and breathe into it 20 times, the effect being that you take back into your lungs the carbon dioxide that you have exhaled. When you breathe in stale or bad air the brain, the automatic centre of control for breathing, calls for deeper breaths, regulating the control of the diaphragm and thus enabling it to break the spasm.

The second practice is even more fun

and works particularly well with susceptible children and adults. Make the victim stand with their arms stretched high above their head whilst you give them sips of water. The exquisite tension created by the certain knowledge that their exposed ribs are a vulnerable target for tickling fingers combined with the effort of trying to breathe calmly and drink at the same time is all too much for any hiccough to survive.

Other Cures to Try

All of these remedies to some extent or another seek to regulate the breathing but some also work on the digestive system. Do be careful how you implement those relying on fright or your victim may end up suffering more than you intended!

- *Cold water or an ice cube* Hold your breath (or hold your nose) whilst drinking a glass of cold water or hold an ice cube in your mouth.
- *Oranges* Eat an orange or drink 2 tablespoons of pure orange juice.
- *Gripe water or dill seeds* Take a good swig of gripe water or chew a few dill seeds.
- *Cinnamon or cloves* Put 3 drops of the oil of either herb on a sugar lump. Hold it in your mouth until it dissolves then slowly swallow.
- *Shock* A cold key, the large type rather than Yale, should be slipped down the back of the neck or an unexpected thump administered between the shoulder blades! Indeed any kind of shock or fright should do the trick.
- *Holding your breath* Hold for a count of 20.
- *Sneezing* Induce an attack of sneezing. Some sources recommend a feather under the nose, others suggest snuff.
- *Charcoal* At one time it was sug-

gested that charcoal straight from the bonfire was the answer but a charcoal tablet taken with cold water is the modern solution.

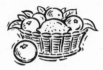

SICKNESS

To everything there is a reason and there is always a reason for nausea and vomiting – an infection, poisoning, stress, among others. Until you have managed to pinpoint the cause here is one piece of advice given to me years ago: go to bed, drink plenty and if you want to be sick, be sick, for it is nature's own way of ridding the body of unwanted matter. For any tummy upsets from gastro-enteritis to salmonella or stress add 1 teaspoon of salt to 2 litres(3½ pints) of water and drink in small quantities throughout the day. Do not take food, sugar or aspirins which might exacerbate the condition. Apple cider vinegar or lemon juice in warm water may help if you feel that the problem lies in something that you have eaten. If the feeling is one of general queasiness take a soothing brew of camomile, mint and catnip tea. Hot water with ground cloves or nutmeg are old-fashioned revivers and so are charcoal biscuits, better by far than placing a raw onion on the stomach. If you are not sure why you feel sick try simmering a pinch of freshly grated ginger root with a few leaves of basil in a mug of hot water for 10 minutes, after which time it will either kill or cure.

- *Tarragon wine* Crush 25g(1oz) of fresh tarragon leaves and place them in a jar with 1 stick of vanilla, 150g(6oz) sugar and 600ml (1 pint) of brandy. Leave to macerate for one month on a warm windowsill, shaking daily. Strain, bottle and keep for curing nausea in emergencies.

Travellers' Comforts

Travel sickness – giddiness, nausea and headaches – may be caused by the movement of any vehicle from a Rolls Royce to a roller coaster. Modern remedies suggest taking vitamin B_6 before a journey to calm the nerves, hypnosis and acupuncture to cure sea sickness, diverting children's attention from the possibility of being sick by game-playing (but do not read in a moving vehicle), and suspending a small chain from the back of the car in which you are travelling, a remedy which I find also requires suspending disbelief. One cure which works is Dr Bach's Rescue Remedy and so too do the following.

Suck a slice of lemon or a piece of ginger root or sip tincture of ginger in hot water. Valerian pastilles or tea are useful too.

Press just below the wrist with three fingers and take deep breaths.

On a sea journey take hot sweet tea and gingerbread for the children and Whisky Mac in moderation for yourself. Do not go below deck unless absolutely necessary.

On any journey do not give children orange juice and chocolate. This fatal combination will cause the most stalwart child to throw up.

FOOD AND ALCOHOL POISONING

It has to be stressed that everybody should have a working knowledge of which berries and plants are poisonous and if anything dubious is swallowed it is essential that you get to a hospital immediately. The same applies to pills or household cleansers that might be swallowed or are suspected of having been swallowed by a child. It does not matter if you are wrong – just dial 999 immediately.

The taste in your mouth and instant queasiness may tell you that you have eaten bad food. The old-fashioned remedy to clear the stomach of something unpleasant was to swallow a strong solution of salt or mustard water followed by castor oil after the former had been expelled. Stewed fennel, the leaves of horseradish or a strong dose of apple cider vinegar have all been utilized in a bid to clear the stomach of bad food and many people swear by 2 tablespoons of olive oil as an emergency measure. However for those people who have managed to poison themselves with an excess of alcohol (which is not to be confused with a hangover), give them lots and lots of water and keep them upright, awake and moving. When they have returned to some semblance of consciousness – and then only – administer weak black coffee, dry toast and vitamin B or yeast tablets and keep the patient walking.

In times past those at risk of being poisoned by their enemies ate great quantities of figs pounded with hazelnuts as a preventative.

● *Half a pint of vegetable oil* I have seen this remedy poured down the throat of someone who was suspected of having eaten a toadstool when they were far from home and far from help. The results were spectacular and it is recommended as an antidote in most situations when you cannot identify the poison or cannot immediately reach an emergency service.

Bowel Disorders

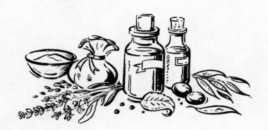

Constipation

The most common causes of constipation are a poor diet, stress or the lack of exercise and fresh air. Constipation not only leads to a general feeling of malaise but because the body becomes toxic can actually cause or exacerbate many ailments, including thumping headaches, spots, hypertension, heartburn, catarrh, arthritis and rheumatism. It can also make you extremely bad tempered. The simplest answer is to ensure that you eat a high-fibre diet including fresh fruit and vegetables, particularly apples, pears and strong greenstuffs, plenty of live yoghurt and drink lots of fresh water. Cut down on refined foods, red meat, coffee and tea. Particularly avoid convenience and junk foods.

One of the most frequent causes of pallid listlessness and 'tummy ache' in children is constipation and an important thing to remember is not to allow them to become reliant on laxatives but to form the habit of their going to the lavatory at a regular time each day whether or not they consider it to be a waste of time.

The oldest and simplest suggestions for a regular movement of the bowels varied from taking a glass of cold water morning and night, conversely, taking a hot drink and a pipeful of tobacco after breakfast. Cold baths daily vied in popularity with the 15-second icy cold sitz bath, whilst gentler souls fell back on the old standby of a spoonful of honey each morning or the ever-faithful 'apple a day'. Genteel nursery nurses and sterner nannies resorted to the well-tried rose petal jelly or home-made syrup of figs, both of which were preferable to chewing the searing mustard leaf or inflicting the enema of red hot chilli pepper seeds much favoured by the native Indians of certain South American countries – a remedy which I am bound to say probably did more to kill than to cure.

Gentle Aperients for Children

Rose Petal Jelly
100g(4oz) white rose petals
1 tablespoon lemon juice
2 tablespoons orange juice
2 tablespoons clear honey
450g(1lb) white cane sugar
150ml(¼ pint) water

Cut the base from the petals and discard them. Place all the ingredients except the petals in a stainless steel pan with a heavy base and leave to stand without heat until the sugar has dissolved. Add the rose petals and heat very gently then continue to cook in this very slow fashion, stirring constantly, until the petals appear to dissolve. Allow the mixture to cool a little before potting. Seal when cold. What you will have is a wobbly syrup with transparent pieces of petal floating in it. Taken by the teaspoon it is a gentle laxative and it is also an effective remedy for tonsillitis.

● *Elderflower tea* Deliciously perfumed, it probably does more to make a fractious child feel cosseted and relax.
● *Peach blossom drink* One teaspoon of dried peach blossoms infused in a cup of boiling milk and drunk twice daily has got to be far more acceptable to a child than some things that I can think of.

A Liquorice Tea
100g(4oz) liquorice root
1 litre(1¾ pints) water
pinch of mallow flowers
honey

Chop the root and put it in a stainless steel pan with the water. Bring to the boil and simmer for 15 minutes. Cover and leave to steep overnight then strain before using. Heat 1 cup as it is needed, infusing a pinch of mallow flowers in it for 10 minutes before drinking. Sweeten with honey and take first thing in the morning when needed.

Syrup of Figs I
50g(2oz) dried figs
50g(2oz) raisins
50g(2oz) barley
1.5 litres(2⅔ pints)
15g(½oz) liquorice root, chopped

Bring the fruit, barley and water to the boil then simmer, covered, for 15 minutes. Add the chopped liquorice then cover and leave to stand overnight. Strain, bottle and keep in the refrigerator. Take 1 tablespoon when needed. Children find this less aggressive in both flavour and result than most of the other concoctions mentioned in this chapter.
● *Liquorice sweets* These are effective but make sure that teeth are well brushed afterwards.
● *Rosemary, hyssop, fennel, marjoram or camomile oil* A child will feel a lot happier when its poor wretched tummy is given a soothing rub with a sweetly scented oil. A few drops of any of these essential oils diluted with sunflower or olive oil will relieve tension and encourage bowel movement when rubbed gently into the abdomen. A drop or two of camphor may be used in conjunction with another oil.

Sterner Measures

Syrup of Figs II
25g(1oz) senna pods
600ml(1 pint) boiling water
225g(8oz) dried prunes
1 litre(1¾ pints) cold water
225g(8oz) dried figs
4 tablespoons blackstrap molasses

Steep the senna pods in the boiling water for 20 minutes then strain. Place the prunes in a bowl large enough to accommodate their swelling and cover with the cold water. Leave overnight. The next day cook both fruits in the prune water until soft then strain, reserving the liquor. Chop the fruit, discarding the stones, and return the chopped fruit, the fruity liquor, the senna tea and the molasses to the pan and simmer until thick and soft. Pour into warm, dry jars and seal when cold. Take at night in the quantities of 1 tablespoon for adults or 2 teaspoons for children. This recipe originated with the matron of one of our better known public schools where it was unlovingly referred to as 'Gunpowder'.

- *Castor oil and orange juice* One tablespoon of each mixed together and taken at night is better than liquid paraffin or cascara.
- *Salts* From Glauber's and Carlsbad to Andrews and Epsom, these are all effective.
- *Olive oil* One teaspoon of olive oil or any good vegetable oil taken each morning will lubricate the system.
- *Bran* Two teaspoons daily may at first have a dramatic effect but taken every morning, sprinkled on cereal, will ensure a regular movement. Small children may be given a little on the tip of a spoon.

- *Blackstrap molasses* Full of vitamin B, take it in milk, fruit juice or water.
- *Honey and hot water* Use in the proportions of 1 teaspoon to 1 cup of hot water.
- *Lemon and honey* Squeeze the juice of ½ lemon into hot water with a pinch of sea salt and 1 teaspoon of honey.
- *Slippery elm* Mix the powdered bark to a drink with warm water and honey.
- *Iceland moss* Sip the water from gently cooked Iceland moss.
- *Agar-agar* This gelatinous substance made from seaweed is rich in minerals and was at one time a popular health food. It is a good gentle laxative and can be used to make slightly cloudy jellies or sprinkled into other foods such as soup. In vegetarian and vegan cookery it is commonly used to replace animal-derived gelatine.

Diet and Drink

- *Prunes and figs* As tradition relates, both these dried fruits have amazingly laxative properties and are delicious eaten as they are. However, if you wish to cook them place them in a deep bowl, cover with boiling water and leave to stand overnight. Drink the liquid and eat the fruit first thing in the morning.
- *Plain live yoghurt* Children will need no encouragement to eat these two very pleasant breakfast dishes: apricots mashed with honey and mixed into a bowl of yoghurt; shredded raw apple, honey and yoghurt with or without a sprinkling of bran.
- *Rhubarb* Stew with honey then eat or drink the juice from the cooked fruit every morning.
- *Baked potato in its jacket* Eaten plain, including the skin, this will relieve constipation and is also remarkably effective in easing migraine.

• *Apples* As well as taking the popular 'apple a day' use them in salads and desserts. The following is a particularly good recipe as horseradish has a cleansing and purifying effect on the system.

Apple with Horseradish
1 crisp eating apple
½ teaspoon freshly grated horseradish
lemon juice
1 tablespoon yoghurt or sour cream

Grate the apple and mix it with the remaining ingredients.

• *Fruit and vegetable juices* If it is possible to make your own from fresh produce do so and drink immediately for maximum benefit.

• *Carrots* Eaten raw they add valuable minerals and vitamins to the diet. Also try this nourishing soup which is sweet and tasty enough to tempt children and acts as a mild aperient.

Carrot Soup
1 onion, chopped
2 cloves garlic, chopped
2 tablespoons olive oil
6 carrots, thinly sliced
¼ bulb fennel, thinly sliced
fresh thyme and bay leaf
sea salt
300ml(½ pint) chicken stock
300ml(½ pint) warmed milk
parsley to garnish

Fry the onion and garlic gently in the olive oil until soft. Add the carrots and fennel and toss lightly until golden brown. Add the herbs, seasoning and stock, cover and simmer until the vegetables are soft. Discard the bay leaf then purée the mixture. Return to the pan and heat through adding as much of the warmed milk as is necessary to give you the right consistency. Garnish with plenty of chopped parsley and serve with wholemeal bread.

Wholewheat and Bran Bread
1.5kg(3½lb) wholemeal flour
3 tablespoons bran
1 tablespoon sea salt
40g(1½oz) dried yeast
4 tablespoons molasses or treacle
1.25 litres(2¼ pints) water

Put the flour, bran and salt into a large bowl and stand in a warm oven. Mix together the yeast, molasses and 150ml(¼ pint) of the water warmed to blood heat. Leave to stand in a warm place for about five minutes, when it should be spongy. Grease four 450g(1lb) loaf tins and put them to warm. Stir the yeast mixture well and pour it into the centre of the flour adding the remainder of the warmed water. Using your hand incorporate the flour from the sides of the bowl into the yeast mixture and continue kneading until you have a wettish dough. Divide equally among the tins, cover loosely with a cloth and leave in a warm, draught-free spot for 20 minutes to rise. Preheat the oven to 230°C/450°F/gas mark 8. When the loaves have risen by about one third pop them into the oven and bake for 40 minutes. They should be well browned and sound faintly hollow when tapped on the bottom.

DIARRHOEA

Judging by the number of ancient remedies which abound world-wide for this horrid affliction, diarrhoea appears to have been a major problem since the beginning of time, presumably as a result of man eating things which he should not have eaten or which were either contaminated or had gone bad. Infection was also carried through inadequate water supplies and drainage systems whilst health and hygiene in the home was fairly scanty.

The long-term or chronic condition of diarrhoea is usually found to be caused by one of the following: a poor or inadequate diet; consistently eating foodstuffs to which one is unknowingly allergic; cooking foods in aluminium pans over a long period of time; perpetual emotional dramas or stress. Those acute griping attacks which usually last for no longer than 24 hours may be caused by one of the following: an infection from contaminated food or water, in some cases by antibiotics, over eating, an excess of sugar, stress or fright (you have heard the expression 'one's bowels turning to water'). Children, particularly babies, are also vulnerable to a change of diet or milk, teething and, strangely enough, sultry weather.

The majority of people who suffer from acute attacks of diarrhoea usually do so abroad and this is borne out by the list of names given to the problem ranging from 'Tangiers trot' to 'cruise blues'. Unaccustomed food, different water, too much sun, too much alcohol and quite frequently too much of everything else, including stress, leads to gyppy tummy. Egypt does seem to be the one place where no stomach is safe and the only person I know of who survived unscathed ate all the highly spiced foods but no salads, drank neat whisky and cleaned his teeth in gin. According to scientists, water does not have to be contaminated to make you ill: it is quite enough that it is different and that the body is unused to it.

Centuries ago men knew when and where not to gather certain foodstuffs. Wild rabbits were not caught at certain times of the year for the flesh would be contaminated by the plants they had eaten. Mussels were not picked from wood beneath the water but only from rocks. Smallholders never fed offal to their chickens or meat scraps to their pigs. Nuts, berries, fruit, vegetables, fish and meat were eaten only within their natural seasons, not only because they were unavailable at other times but to protect the supply and to ensure that the conditions were right in which to keep them for as long as possible without adverse effect. Nowadays, due to modern farming, collection and storage methods, we have overcome most of these barriers but in doing so have created many other problems.

Instant Relief

Although the desire to stop a painful attack of diarrhoea may appear to be of paramount importance it is better to allow the body to flush itself clean of the cause completely, which will usually take about 24 hours. However, if it continues over 48 hours professional advice should be sought. Do not delay with young children: if a gentle remedy has not been effective within 12 hours seek advice. The same applies to babies. If it is not the normal result expected due to teething, or the introduction of new foods or bottle feeding, for example, seek help as soon as possible.

Eat very little when the tummy is badly upset, keeping the consumption down to bland, dry foods and lots of water. Eat only light meals during recovery and do not tempt providence. If it is a case of real emergency, such as travelling home from holiday and being confined to coach or plane or an important meeting which just cannot be put off, try either kaolin and morphine or J. Collis Brown's Mixture. They are both patent medicines which are very old-fashioned and effective, but do refer to the instruction for dosage and suitability for children. Most of the old wives' remedies are as useful today as they were yesterday but pity the poor sailor who had little choice between chewing tarred rope or his bottle of rum.

Long-Term Settlers

- *Drink plenty* Dehydration is the most acute problem arising from a severe attack of diarrhoea so drink lots of fresh, clear water. If you are far from home buy a well known mineral water. Alternatively experts recommend making up quantities of the following: 1 litre($1\frac{3}{4}$ pints) of freshly boiled mineral water, 2 tablespoons of honey, $\frac{1}{4}$ teaspoon of sea salt, $\frac{1}{4}$ teaspoon of bicarbonate of soda and a little fresh lemon juice. Adults should take a little every five minutes until at least 3 litres($5\frac{1}{4}$ pints) have been consumed within a 24 hour period. Children will only need to drink 1 litre($1\frac{3}{4}$ pints) and the very young even less. This is an invaluable remedy if sickness strikes abroad but do use a reliable brand of water that has been 'bottled at source'.
- *Barley water* The most reliable and old fashioned standby, make it up with or without lemon.
- *Arrowroot or slippery elm* Mix 1 tablespoon of either powder to a paste with a little cold water then thin to a gruel with boiling water. Add honey and cinnamon to taste. Children can also take this but use only 1 teaspoon of the powder.
- *Rice* A good food for a child who is suffering is plain boiled white rice mashed up with bananas.
- *Rice water* Boil 25g(1oz) of rice gently in 1 litre($1\frac{3}{4}$ pints) of water for $1\frac{1}{2}$

hours. Strain and drink the liquid to soothe the irritated bowel.
- *Oats* Make a thin gruel with oatmeal or a handful of raw oats.
- *Plain live yoghurt* This will kill off unwanted bacteria.
- *Leeks* Cook 8 good-sized well-washed leeks in 2 litres($3\frac{1}{2}$ pints) of water for three hours in a covered pan. A teaspoon of the resulting liquid drunk every five minutes will relieve diarrhoea in children.
- *Potato juice* The juice of fresh potatoes mixed with carrot juice and honey clears the bowels of infection. However 'green' potatoes, which are those which have been exposed to light, are very dangerous when eaten raw. Potatoes which have been cooked and left for over 24 hours before eating are also a prime cause of illness, so do not keep them for bubble and squeak but throw them away.
- *Pomegranate juice* Crush the flesh to extract the juice and drink a spoonful at a time regularly throughout the day. This is a remedy from Egypt, where they know about such things!
- *Grape juice* If an allergic reaction to a food or drug is the cause of sickness and diarrhoea drink 2 glasses of grape juice and water.

Store Cupboard Remedies

- *Sloes* These are a very ancient medicine for an upset stomach and combined with gin they leave little else to be desired.

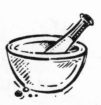

Sloe Gin

a quantity of fat black sloes picked
after the first frost
1 bottle gin
white cane sugar

Wash the sloes thoroughly and prick them through with a needle to release the juices. Drink a third of the gin and if you are still in any fit state continue thus. Put enough sloes in the bottle to reach a third of the way up. If you have a sweet tooth add 4 tablespoons of sugar but if you are an aesthetic drinker or are making this for purely medicinal purposes 2 tablespoons will suffice. Seal tightly and shake every day for three months, by which time the sloes should have nicely macerated.

● *Blackberries* The root, the leaf and particularly the pippy fruit are all taken in one way or another to remedy diarrhoea and I find this cordial is particularly pleasant tasting and soothing for fractious children of all ages, to say nothing of fractious adults. It is certainly much nicer than the other alcoholic recipe of moss boiled in red wine.

Blackberry Cordial

1 litre(1¾ pints) home-made
blackberry juice
450g(1lb) cane sugar or 225g(8oz)
mild-flavoured honey
1 teaspoon each ground cloves,
cinnamon and nutmeg
150ml(¼ pint) brandy

Boil together the blackberry juice and the sugar or honey, stirring well until dissolved. Continue to boil until a syrup has formed then remove from the heat, skim and add the spices. Stir well and bring to the boil then continue to simmer for about 20 minutes. Remove from the heat and allow to settle before straining through a muslin cloth into a hot jug. While the cordial is still very hot add the brandy, stir well and pour into heat-resistant bottles, stopping at 2cm(¾ inch) from the top. Seal with screw-top lids, giving a half turn back to allow for expansion. Stand the bottles on a wire rack in a large pan, making sure that they do not touch. Fill up the pan with very hot water past the level of the cordial in the bottles and bring to the boil. Boil for five to eight minutes. Remove the bottles from the pan and place them on a wooden board or a cloth. Tighten the lids immediately. Take in the quantities of 1 tablespoon in 1 wineglass of hot water.

Quick Comforters

● *Oil of peppermint* Take a few drops in hot water.
● *Warm water and honey* A small cup is an ideal soother for small children.
● *Port and brandy* This mixture warms and settles the stomach and, provided you are not nauseous, makes you feel so much better.
● *Cayenne pepper* One teaspoon stirred into a glass of hot water and swallowed quickly is incredibly disinfectant, if you can bear to take it. So is hot curry but this may well have been the cause of your downfall in the first place.
● *Camomile, sage, meadowsweet, peppermint or catnip* A very mild infusion of any one of these herbs is suitable for small children. Camomile is particularly useful for babies who have tummy trouble caused by teething. Adults will also benefit from a stronger tea.
● *Rose hip syrup* Take in hot water after first making sure than an excess of vitamin C is not the original cause of the problem.

• *Red clover syrup* (see recipe on page 114) is also good for diarrhoea.

• *Massage* A gentle massage of the abdomen will reduce the ache caused by this type of tummy upset which children find particularly distressing. Use 1 tablespoon of warm sunflower oil with several drops of one of the following essential oils added to give extra benefit: geranium, lavender, peppermint, sage, clove or garlic.

• *Warm compresses* Another old-fashioned idea was to use a compress of leeks but I think that a much nicer idea is to use a warm compress of camomile tea.

• *Onion* Peel and slice a large onion and leave to infuse in a covered bowl with 1 litre(1¾ pints) water. The liquid is then drunk by the cup. This is also an excellent remedy for babies and small children if it is sweetened with honey and given by the small teaspoonful. The juice from raw onion on the hands makes a first-class disinfectant when dealing with children who have diarrhoea, especially when changing nappies or cleaning potties.

• *Milky beverages* A red-hot poker immersed for 30 seconds in a cup of boiling milk was believed to impart iron emanations to the drink. You may prefer a teaspoon of cinnamon or allspice in warm milk, both of which are warming and antiseptic.

WORMS

Not the garden variety but the intestinal parasite, round and tapeworm, are a subject which causes more than just a frisson of embarrassment in today's hygienic society yet suffering from worms was, only a brief time ago, a very common ailment. Therefore many of the old-fashioned remedies do still work very well.

Old-fashioned Remedies

All the following must be taken first thing in the morning.

• *Lemons* Crush lemon pips in honey and take by the teaspoon or make a strong brew of pure lemon juice and crushed thyme.

• *Thyme* Dice 1 tablespoon of the fresh stem into tiny pieces and simmer for 10 minutes in 150ml(¼ pint) of fresh barley water.

• *Watermelon seeds* Simmer a good handful of seeds in water until a thick concoction is obtained.

• *Pumpkin seeds* Crushed with milk and honey and taken before breakfast for three consecutive days was the accepted remedy for tapeworm. The Nice Breakfast food (page 152) eaten every day will undoubtedly ensure that this problem does not arise.

• *Cabbage juice* Take 4 tablespoons of freshly extracted cabbage juice every morning for three days.

• *Liquorice* A dose of liquorice after a dose of salts then fasting for four hours might, I feel, be a somewhat explosive remedy.

• *Basil or tansy* Chew basil leaves daily or drink tansy tea to ensure that worms do not thrive.

• *Garlic* Taken regularly garlic will ensure that the problem does not arise but if it should do so then you could follow the old-fashioned cure of chewing several garlic cloves at night and using a garlic clove as a suppository. However, rather than inflict this uncomfortable cure upon one's family I suggest chewing the garlic as directed and using instead a little garlic ointment smeared around the anus every night for a fortnight. This will also ensure that one is not bitten on the bottom by a vampire.

KIDNEY TROUBLES

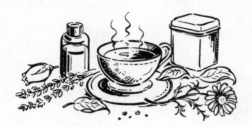

FEELING SLUGGISH

We are in the habit, much to the medical profession's annoyance, of attributing every unaccustomed twinge and pain from backache to headache and nausea to 'a bit of trouble with the kidneys'. Problems affecting the kidneys, especially if·it is an inability to pass water or the searing pain of cystitis, are a matter for professional advice and the remedies below are given purely to bring comfort and relief if you are feeling sluggish and low with that unpleasant feeling that your body needs a good 'de-coke'.

Cleansing the System

● *Honey, hot water and lemon juice* Taken every morning and night this will act as a deterrent to kidney and liver problems.
● *Watercress, parsley, grapes and runner beans* Eat plenty of these which are especially beneficial if you are prone to gravel.

Have lots and lots to drink but not too much tea and coffee which will only make you feel more sluggish. Barley water or just water are hard to beat.
● *Cranberry juice* Drink a 225ml(8 fl oz) glass every morning.
● *Melon, pumpkin and marrow* The flesh of melon, the seeds of pumpkin and the juice of marrow all act as purifiers. A tea made from watermelon pips was considered an excellent remedy for women who found their bladders to be weak after childbirth.
● *Asparagus* Eat plenty of asparagus as it is a good diuretic.
● *Dandelion tea and leaves* Dandelion is a marvellous tonic. Try also the Excellent Salad described under **Liver Disorders** and add plenty of chopped chives for extra benefit.
● *Strawberry juice* Strain to remove the pips and drink with plenty of mineral water.

- *Parsnips* Both the vegetable and the juice are recommended.
- *Mangoes* These were used by expatriates in the far-flung corners of our one-time Empire to remedy kidney problems caused by an excess of alcohol.
- *Cardoon* This large thistle very similar to the globe artichoke is used as a powerful diuretic to remedy kidney and liver disorders.
- *Sloes* Their juice or the water in which they have been cooked will help dispel cystitis and gravel and improve the working of the kidneys.

KIDNEY STONES

Kidney stones, usually quite minute, are a more common problem than people realize but they make themselves felt as they are being expelled from the body. A sharp pain in the side, lower back or abdomen over a period of days or weeks may denote the presence of kidney stones and you should seek professional advice to ensure that they do not cause damage to the kidneys. Except in dire circumstances a physician will usually recommend that they be allowed to disperse naturally. In the meantime drink large quantities of water and consider the following.

Drinks to Soothe and Cure

- *Beetroot* Beet tops and beetroot taken daily is an old-fashioned suggestion for dissolving kidney stones.

A Tea to Relieve Kidney Pains
25g(1oz) each grated asparagus root, fennel bulb, parsley root and celery
600ml(1 pint) boiling water

Cover the grated vegetables and herbs with the water and leave to stand for 10 minutes. Strain and serve with a dash of lemon juice. Drink 1 small glass before meals for 3 days when discomfort is felt.

- *Burdock, tansy, dandelion, marsh mallow root and urva ursi* Mix together 25g(1oz) of each and take 1 teaspoon in 1 cup of boiling water to disperse gravel.
- *Nettles and tansy* Add 1 handful of each of the fresh herbs to 1 litre(1¾ pints) of water. Boil for 10 minutes and drink a small cupful every four hours.
- *Linseed* Boil 4 tablespoons of linseed in 1 litre(1¾ pints) of water then strain and drink the liquid with lemon and honey. It will soothe all kidney disorders.
- *Sweetcorn* A tea made with the silky tassels from the sweetcorn cob is a very old-fashioned and universal cure for irritations of the urinary tract.
- *Glycerine* Take 1 tablespoon of glycerine on an empty stomach.
- *Parsley piert* This plant was known as 'break stone' to the old-fashioned herbalist. Take 25g(1oz) in 600ml(1 pint) of boiling water.
- *Kill or cure* My French brother-in-law dispersed his kidney stones by drinking daily several glasses of his own rough Norman cider.

BEDWETTING

Most parents will have had a child wetting the bed and once the child is of an age to know better this becomes an infrequent occurrence, only happening when they are ill or unhappy.

Occasionally it is caused by a child being a very heavy sleeper or as a result of pressure on the bladder. In the latter case, if it persists, professional advice should be taken for reassurance as there may be a long-standing and unnoticed problem. It is my opinion that the worst thing you can do when a child wets the bed is to make a fuss and blow up the whole thing out of proportion which will only exacerbate the problem. Many people believe that bedwetting has its cause in a lack of calcium and magnesium so ensure that plenty of good greenstuff, milk and yoghurt are included in the diet. Avoid refined foods and additives, particularly 'junk foods'.

Children need a lot of exercise, both physical and mental, but they do not need problems and if you think that a nasty niggling worry is at the bottom of this minor disaster try to get your child to tell you about it. Attention at night-time, a story, a small game and plenty of kisses and cuddles to reassure may be tiring and time-consuming but they are far less so and far more rewarding than washing sheets. However as a last resort a rubber sheet under the bedlinen to protect the mattress is a better alternative than the old-fashioned, beastly devices of tying a bandage around the child's chest with a big knot in it to ensure a restless sleep or waking the child every hour or so to insist that they spend a penny which really can institute a major problem. One remedy which does appear to work very well on children is to massage the areas of the kidneys and lower abdomen with warm olive oil before bed. It is a very old-fashioned and successful idea.

Exercise

Both adults and children should exercise a little before bedtime to relieve pressure on the bladder. Some Yoga positions are designed specifically to achieve this.

Drinks

It is obviously foolhardy to give bedtime drinks to a child who wets the bed. Nevertheless soothing possets given half an hour beforehand will ensure dreamless sleep: it may be that nightmares, especially the ones which they cannot remember, are the problem. Make sure they spend a penny before tucking in.

- *Hot milk*   A small cup of hot milk with honey and cinnamon is simple and soothing.
- *Infusion of sweetcorn and honey*   As in the case of asparagus and golden rod tea (both of which are recommended) this remedy should only be taken well in advance of bedtime. St John's wort and plantain made into a small tea will also help. Adults should take lady's mantle tea.
- *Cream of tartar*   Dissolve 1 teaspoon in 500ml(1 pint) of boiling water and sweeten with honey and lemon. Take by the small glass. This could possibly be preferable to Epsom salts but both may be especially effective when constipation is causing the problem.
- *A long-term remedy*   Take 15g(½oz) of nettle seeds and 50g(2oz) of fresh rye flour, pound them to a paste with honey and form into small cakes. Bake them in a low oven until cooked. Eat one every evening until the problem stops which should be no longer than three weeks.

CYSTITIS

This is a very uncomfortable and painful condition caused by inflammation of the bladder. The symptoms are an aching pain in the lower back and abdomen and the most fiery pain when passing water. The inflammation and infection may pass to the kidneys so you must seek professional advice. If you receive antibiotics in treatment you would be well advised to eat a large pot of plain live yoghurt daily as a precaution against vaginal thrush. Although too much over enthusiastic lovemaking can cause cystitis it is not a 'social disease' but is often the result of a bad catarrhal infection, kidney stones or hormone pills. Whatever the cause, warmth and rest are essential.

Soothing Essential Oils

You will probably feel so miserable if you are suffering from cystitis that the kindest remedy is a warm bath to which you have added a few drops of oil of pine. To further pamper yourself and help bring about a cure a few drops of cedarwood oil should be rubbed into the lower abdomen. A trick taught me when I was pregnant and very dubious about taking any 'drugs' was to make up the following: a few drops each of essential oil of juniper, pine, parsley and sandalwood in a cup of sunflower oil. This I rubbed into my lower abdomen (when I could find it), my lower back and, amazingly, the backs of my knees. Finally hop into a warm bed and keep a well-wrapped hot water bottle against the backs of the knees.

Drinks to Bring Relief

● *Water* Drink lots of tepid water – not before, not during but after you have made love if you are prone to cystitis.
● *Chervil, horsetail, shepherd's purse and birch leaf* A tea of any one of these herbs will bring relief.

● *Bilberry leaves* Infuse 25g(1oz) of bilberry leaves in 1 litre(1¾ pints) of boiling water for 15 minutes. Drink 2 or 3 cups daily to ease the pain of cystitis.
● *Potato water* Drink the water from boiled potatoes. (Do not cook them in an aluminium saucepan.)
● *Sweetcorn* Make a tea from the silky tassels of the cob and also eat the fresh vegetable.
● *Cherry stalks and peach leaf tea* One teaspoon of each in 600ml(1 pint) of water soothes considerably. Cherry stalks were at one time used as a diuretic.
● *Cherries* As well as the stalks, the fruit themselves are good for you. If you often suffer from kidney disorders and cystitis frequently recurs make this delicious syrup and drink by the tablespoon.

Cherry Syrup
500g(1lb) cherries (preferably a cooking variety)
175ml(6 fl oz) water
unrefined cane sugar

Wash the cherries, keeping their stalks on, and put them into a double boiler with the water. Cook gently until the fruit is very soft, helping the process along with a little judicious mashing with a wooden spoon, if necessary. Crush a few of the stones and add the kernels to the pan. When the cherries are pulpy strain them through a muslin cloth, squeezing out every last drop of juice. Measure the liquid and for every 500ml(1 pint) take 250g(8oz) of sugar. Put both in a saucepan and heat gently, stirring well, until the sugar has dissolved. Boil gently to a syrupy consistency and bottle in a dry, hot container. Seal tightly. It will keep for quite a long time if refrigerated.

● *Marsh mallow* A decoction of marsh mallow is often used to help you 'spend a penny'. However in this case it is used to offset the effects of taking antibiotics: 1 teaspoon of marsh mallow root to 1 cup of boiling water, left to stand for five minutes and then sweetened with honey.

Liver Disorders

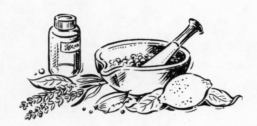

Liver ailments include gallstones, jaundice, hepatitis and biliousness.

Gaze deeply into any romantic Frenchman's eyes and ask him from whence spring his tenderest emotions and you will be disappointed when, breathing garlic and red wine lustily upon you, he admits to it being his liver rather than his heart. This is not surprising for without the proper functioning of this vital organ no self-respecting Frenchman can enjoy his food – that other basic fundamental of his life – and it is usually as a result of an excess in this area that the poor old liver does falter. Tradition has it that coffee, red wine, brandy and rich foods all contribute to a sluggish liver and the resulting queasiness and jaundiced outlook on life when we do not seem to be feeling at our best. That is the liverishness for which Mr Carter used to make his Little Liver Pills.

Sensible suggestions for improving this state of affairs are numerous: cut out coffee and tea, eat more fruit and vegetables, drink plenty of soda water or sparkling mineral water (hence the popularity of Perrier in France), eat more garlic, take more exercise. The very nicest of them all is to enjoy a good laugh every morning when you rise from bed.

A Cleansing Approach

Fast for two days taking only many glasses of sparkling mineral water with the juice of ½ lemon squeezed into each. Pick a weekend or a time when you will be fairly inactive.

• Try a diet of grapes only for one day or more if necessary. They do cleanse the system wonderfully well.
• Take garlic capsules daily.
• When feeling really out of sorts drink only water and apple juice every two hours.
• *Green cocktail, sunset slinger* Take either of these by the wineglass daily (see pages 77 and 53). Alternatively mix together equal quantities of carrot, beetroot and celery juice.

• *An excellent salad* Prepare yourself a large plateful of beetroot, radish, dandelion leaves, chicory, fennel and artichoke.

• *Apple cider vinegar or pure lemon juice* Add 1 teaspoon to a small wineglass of warm water with a very little honey and take every three hours as needed.

• *Dandelion and hops* A tea made with equal parts of each is very therapeutic and drinkable. So are fennel, tansy, agrimony and camomile teas.

• *Lettuce* Brew up several good green lettuce leaves and drink daily.

• *Angelica* Chew angelica as a digestive – but not last thing at night or it could stop you sleeping.

GALLSTONES

The most obviously painful of the conditions associated with the liver and the gall bladder, gallstones are first recognized by sharp pains in the side and chest, a feeling of distention and discomfort, general queasiness and a tendency to biliousness. There is no doubt that if you have these symptoms you will seek professional advice and there is no doubt that if you are fat, female and over 40 you will be diagnosed as having gallstones. It therefore comes as something of a relief to know that this chauvinistic attitude is now considered misplaced but nevertheless a poor diet leading to excess weight, little exercise and a disposition to harbour ill will or to become stressed do encourage the formation of gallstones. Those phrases which trip off the tongue – 'it galls me', 'as bitter as gall' – all relate to an unhappy frame of mind and these negative emotions have a physical result in that they stop the bile flowing freely. The old-fashioned cure for this was for the victim to drink a ½

pint of olive oil at one intake thus stimulating the gall bladder to secrete bile which would take small stones with it. It also kept your mind on other things!

Diet

A regular intake of artichokes, asparagus, kelp and barley water is to be preferred to the remedy which might have been used a century or less ago of nine lice eaten on bread. These were supposed to make their way straight to the gall bladder where they set to work on the problem. As it was firmly believed that gallstones were caused by fright and would be dispelled by fright, this latter solution must surely have been successful.

Do not take strong purgatives but keep the bowels open by eating plenty of prunes and figs.

Gentle Remedies

• *Olive oil and pure lemon juice* Take 1 tablespoon of each every 15 minutes until 200ml(8 fl oz) of oil and several lemons have been consumed.

• Pack the painful area with warm compresses, poultices or a hot-water bottle. Use Epsom salts in a bath to ease pain.

• *Essential oils of rosemary, nutmeg, lemon, camphor, hyssop and eucalyptus* These can all be used in a carrier oil, to rub the aching area or the soles of the feet. This will relieve stress. Many of the liniments to be found under **Aches and Pains** will also bring relief and warmth.

● *Horseradish* Make the leaves into a tea. Couch grass was also recommended to break up both gallstones and kidney stones.

JAUNDICE

'Jaundiced' is the way you look when you have something wrong with your liver and from the layman's point of view that is the most simple way to explain it. The cause must be investigated by a professional for it may be a symptom of hepatitis or a problem associated with the gall bladder, or it may be the use of certain drugs which has given the yellow hue to the skin and a dingy tinge to the eyes.

Yellow jaundice is not an illness in itself but judging by the remedies suggested for treating it the ancient medics obviously felt that sympathetic medicine in the form of anything golden yellow could be used. These ranged from copious quantities of carrot juice to wormwood, horehound, sheep's dung, ale and rum all stewed up in water and also included all the yellow plants –

amber, gold cloth, walnuts, wormseed and brimstone – after surviving which you could survive anything! One of the medicines prescribed to cure jaundice was a purgative made of camomile, senna, ginger and jalap (from the ipomoea plant) and it is presumably from this source that the slang word for medicine – jollop – arose. You can make yourself feel more comfortable by eating asparagus, globe artichokes and kelp and by drinking a great deal of barley water. You may also add Epsom salts to your bath water to relieve the aches and pains but I do not think that the very ancient remedy of dropping an uncorked bottle of your urine into a stream and waiting hopefully for your yellow appearance to die away as do the waters in the stream will bring much comfort. If you had hepatitis this could be positively antisocial.

One old country remedy involved taking the first milk from the cow after calving and giving it to the patient. Such milk is full of good things not to be found in any other milking so this remedy is not as improbable as it sounds.

Conditions of the Blood and Veins

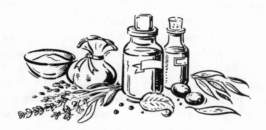

Traditionally there are few conditions of the blood which lend themselves to folklore and its attendant medicines. Anaemia, however, has long been with us and long been recognized.

Anaemia

The symptoms are persistent tiredness, headaches, breathlessness, palpitations, paleness and sometimes depression – probably as a result of the afore-mentioned symptoms. If you feel continually under par in this way seek professional advice as there may be an underlying reason for anaemia. People who are most likely to suffer from the condition are young girls, growing children, women during pregnancy and women who use some forms of contraception. More women than men are affected, primarily because they suffer a more constant blood loss throughout most of their lives.

Although iron deficiency is usually considered to be the main cause of anaemia it may not be due to that alone. Therefore do not treat yourself with large doses of iron (which is the traditional remedy for anaemia) in the form of pills and tonics or you could well end up being disagreeably constipated and headachy. It is more likely that your body is being prohibited from using the iron which is already present by a deficiency of other minerals or vitamins. Lots of strong green vegetables and liver used to be the answer but it is thought more important nowadays to follow a balanced diet overall. Fresh air and walks, which young Victorian ladies would have been instructed to take, certainly improve the supply of oxygen to the blood which is undoubtedly a physical, albeit a temporary improvement. When and if anaemia has been diagnosed and a course of treatment suggested, or if it is found that you are simply suffering from general tiredness and malaise caused by the hassle of everyday affairs, your state of health can only be improved by any of the following old-fashioned and very harmless ideas.

Just a Matter of Diet

The famous 'green cocktail' (see page 77) of spinach, watercress, nettle tops, carrots and beetroot mixed together in a blender to make a 'tonic' juice contains valuable minerals and vitamins. Try it for breakfast or dinner.

Walnuts, sun-dried pears and apricots, raw oats, wheatgerm and pumpkin seeds – what could be nicer than all these ingredients mixed together in a breakfast muesli? All of these foods, together with carrots and beetroot, will improve the general state of health and will also help to restore the good appetite which is usually lacking when fatigue takes over. Sun-dried pears and apricots soaked in red wine and cooked with honey were highly recommended as a breakfast food to tempt the appetite. A glass of aperitif, fortified wine or red wine may also have the same effect.

Most children will baulk at the 'green cocktail' but like carrots so make up instead a good carrot or beetroot soup using the minimum of water to cook the vegetables in. Give them a small glassful of grape juice daily too.

Honey, as always, plays an important part in improving health. Lemon and honey or apple cider vinegar and honey mixed with warm water are good morning or night-time drinks which will help to combat infection when resistance is at a low ebb.

Nettle, chickweed or dandelion tea taken with or without honey are full of valuable minerals and vitamins and are very ancient remedies for debility.

Finally, old-fashioned purists viewing an unresponsively lethargic and listless child often put it down to bloody-minded laziness and enforced a regime of castor oil morning and night to purify the blood. Fresh fruit and vegetables will have a far better long-term effect.

PILES

When we were children and all desperately clamouring to sit on the one radiator in our classroom our teacher would call us to order by informing us that we would give ourselves piles. This is nonsense really because piles are basically caused by constipation, poor circulation, pregnancy, overeating on a low-fibre diet or any circumstance which causes pressure to be put on the veins around the anal passage creating a condition in which they become swollen and twisted. The major problem does seem to be constipation especially of the 'sit and strain' rather than the 'I will wait until I feel like it' variety. Whilst piles may not be caused by sitting on heat I do wonder if they can be cured by the old method of sitting in iced water. The most recommended methods of trying to rid yourself of piles are to eat a high-fibre diet with plenty of bran, take a vitamin B_6 supplement, drink plenty of water and add honey to your diet (some people recommend it as an unguent). Walk whenever you can, every day.

Soothing Suggestions

● *Witch hazel* Keep a bottle of witch hazel in the refrigerator and use it on a cotton wool compress.
● *Garlic or marigold* The old herbalists suggested a suppository of raw garlic cloves, the very thought of which makes

me wince. Garlic oil, cream or skin salve are much more soothing and healing suggestions. Marigold oil or calendula cream are fragrant alternatives.

• *Pilewort (lesser celandine)* This very astringent little herb has been used for many years, as the name implies, to reduce, shrink and soothe piles. A decoction made by simmering 40g(1½oz) of pilewort in ½ litre(scant pint) of water until it is reduced by half can be applied on a hot compress to shrink the swollen veins. Pilewort ointment is the favourite method of application and you can make your own by gathering the roots in the spring. Weigh them and take their weight in fresh lard then pound together. This mixture is left to macerate for five days in a stone jar after which time it is gently heated, strained and pressed through a cloth.

• *Bilberry, sloes or yarrow* Decoctions of any of these are astringent and may also be used on a compress to much the same effect.

• *Blackberry leaf tea* Drink this tea to help the circulation.

• *Roast figs, honey and thyme* Popular as a paste for chilblains, this remedy was also popular as a cure for piles. You may draw the line at the other remedy recommended for both chilblains and piles of 1 tablespoon of honey and glycerine mixed to a fine paste with egg white and flour. However I am assured that it works after one application.

• *Essential oils* Use 1 drop each of myrrh and cypress in 1 dessertspoon of olive oil or 1 drop of geranium oil in cold cream. Cypress oil in hot water can also be used as a soothing compress.

• *Alum and lard* One teaspoon of powdered alum melted into 40g(1½oz) of pure lard is another very old-fashioned remedy.

• *Horse chestnut* Suspend disbelief and carry one in your pocket: as it hardens so will your piles diminish. Another popular belief was to carry a small bag of the root of wood avens around the neck. Why I do not know but sometimes these strange remedies work.

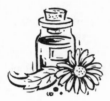

VARICOSE VEINS

We all know what varicose veins look like – the hardened, bulging blue knots standing out in the legs which are caused, some people say, by heredity but which are likely to have been made far worse by neglect. The valves which control the flow of blood in veins and arteries collapse as a result of poor circulation which can be caused by carrying too much weight, especially during pregnancy.

Standing for too many hours at a time is also a prime factor. If you have to stand a lot try to find a few minutes every now and again to take a walk and everybody should make time for a good brisk walk every day.

Sitting on an office chair that is a bad shape can cut off the blood supply particularly if you are overweight, and so can kneeling or sitting with one leg crossed over the other knee. In fact anything that makes a limb 'go to sleep' is bad for it.

Restrictive clothing is another danger. Varicose veins are even less appealing and far more likely to result than a high voice or sterility, so tell that to your son when he buys his next pair of skin-tight denims.

Constipation, smoking and hot baths are all other contributory factors to varicose veins.

Diet

Eat plenty of fruit including grapes, blackcurrants, citrus fruits and rose hips and a regular amount of good green cabbage, spinach, parsley and dandelion. Wheatgerm, brewer's yeast and garlic are further vital elements in the diet.

- *Rosemary tea with honey and elderflower tea* Both of these are old-fashioned remedies to aid the circulation.
- *Bistort tea* Leave 50g(2oz) of bistort root (*Polygonum bistorta* from whose leaves the British used to make Easter Pudding) to macerate in 1 litre(1¾ pints) of cold water for 10 hours. Strain and take 4 cups a day between meals to aid the healing of both varicose veins and piles.

Massage

Rub the legs gently but never scratch varicose veins because the varicose ulcers which may result from a sore place can be very unpleasant indeed.

Wash the legs and massage upwards towards the heart using either witch hazel or tincture of calendula. You may prefer to give the legs alternate hot and cold baths to improve the circulation but you should never, ever take hot baths without splashing the legs in cold water afterwards.

Raise the legs several times a day or sleep with the foot of the bed raised.

Excellent massage oils for varicose veins are olive or, sweet almond oil, the essential oil of cypress (6 drops in the bath or 4 drops in 2 teaspoons of olive oil), calendula, rosemary, lavender or the following. Take equal amounts of oak bark, wild marjoram and walnut leaves. Fill a jar three quarters full with these plants and add enough olive oil to cover. Stand in a double boiler for two hours over a low heat then allow to cool in the pan. Draw off the liquid and pour through a filter.

CHEST INFECTIONS

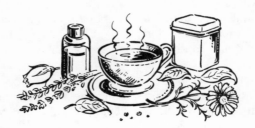

COUGHS

In our relatively safe and hygienic houses and workplaces a cough is likely to be the result of an outside irritant or catarrhal infection, influenza, hayfever or asthma. Although coughs should never be taken lightly, today's remedies are more in the nature of expectorants and soothers to make us more comfortable and to prevent the condition from worsening, whereas in our forefathers' days the onset of a cough might well have indicated the presence of tuberculosis or one of the horrendous occupational diseases which were suffered by so many workers from miners to weavers.

The reason we cough is to rid the surface lining (the mucous membrane) of the throat and upper respiratory tract of an irritation which may be caused by food, smoke, dust particles or excess mucus created by the mucous membrane itself in order to soothe the irritation and inflammation resulting from infection.

Not only is suffering from a cough very aggravating, especially at night, but it is traditionally viewed with alarm as the precursor of something worse and unfortunately inflammation and infection from a head cold can descend to the chest and result in bronchitis or pneumonia if not properly treated. Therefore rather than being suppressed a cough should be soothed, healed and encouraged in order to rid the body of this unwanted mucus, and most old-fashioned and herbal remedies were designed to do just this. If a cough is persistent or if heavily discoloured mucus is 'brought up' professional advice should be sought.

As may be expected, the remedies and advice for curing coughs were legion, ranging from poultices of vinegar and brown paper upon the chest to a fig and liquorice syrup which probably gave the victim other things to think about, and there were plenty of 'robs' and 'toddies' to ensure a good night's sleep. Many remedies, such as saline gargle, were based in sound commonsense although I cannot see how eating dry sugar could have been of benefit unless, in the manner of sucking cough sweets, it was to encourage a flow of soothing saliva which might temporarily ease a tickling cough. However, a syrup of black radish crushed to a pulp with sugar may well have served a nicotined old die-hard and swiftly sought out malingerers but it would have brought tears to the eyes of a child.

It is important for anyone with a cough to drink plenty so make up a good supply of healthy drinks such as lemon barley water, bran tea or oatmeal water and those herbal teas which will act as refreshing and sedative expectorants (see page 117). Fresh fruit and vegetables are very necessary to the diet and are quite often all that anyone suffering from a catarrhal cough will fancy, but bananas, potatoes, nuts and other 'floury' fresh produce should be avoided.

A hot water inhalant is very useful and cider vinegar in hot water is a cheap and cheerful idea which is effective when nothing else is available. It can also be used as a warm compress on the chest – 1 part vinegar to 3 parts hot water. Changed every 15 minutes it will help reduce a wheezy cough.

Cough Syrups

Red Clover Syrup
25g(1oz) fresh red clover blossoms
600ml(1 pint) clear honey
600ml(1 pint) water

Make sure that the flower heads are free from creepy crawlies. Heat the honey and water gently to boiling point and add the blossoms. Simmer for 15 minutes then remove from the heat and leave until cold. Strain through a fine muslin cloth, pressing well to ensure that every drop of delicious syrup is through. Bottle and keep refrigerated. Take 1 or 2 tablespoons as and when needed. Red Clover Syrup is also good for colds and tummy troubles, especially diarrhoea, so it will not be wasted.

Lemon and Glycerine Cough Syrup
juice of 1 lemon
2 tablespoons glycerine
clear honey

Pour the first two ingredients into a 250ml(8 fl oz) capacity jar, stir well and fill up with honey. Seal then shake well and keep refrigrated. Take 1 teaspoonful at a time when needed. This is a good remedy for children who prefer it to the same recipe made with cider vinegar instead of lemon juice.

Garlic Cough Syrup
125ml(4 fl oz) clear honey
1 tablespoon very finely chopped garlic
1 teaspoon very finely grated horseradish

A word of warning before starting: do make sure that the fumes from the horseradish do not waft into your eyes and wash your hands well after preparing, otherwise you may have more problems than a cough to contend with. Mix all the ingredients together in a clean jar and stand them in a pan of hot water placed in a safe, warm place to macerate for one day. Take 1 or 2 teaspoons as needed for a chesty cough (not recommended for children). Diluted with a little warm water it also makes an excellent gargle.

● *Garlic syrup* This is another wonderfully effective old-fashioned remedy made by putting 4 peeled cloves of garlic into a clean jar with 4 tablespoons of clear honey, covering and leaving to stand in a warm place for several hours. The strangely delicious syrup can then be taken 1 teaspoon at a time when needed for bronchial coughs. A regular course of garlic perles will also ensure that coughs are kept at bay.

• *Onion cough syrup* Cut up 6 large, white onions and place them in a double boiler with ½ cup of clear honey. Cover and cook slowly for 2 hours then strain. Take warm at regular intervals to loosen phlegm.

An Old-Fashioned Cough Remedy
100g(4oz) clear honey
100g(4oz) golden syrup
150ml(¼ pint) cider vinegar
6g(⅛oz) paregoric

Mix together with a bone spoon and take three times a day or when coughing.

• *Red cabbage (Boerhaave syrup)* Put the leaves of a red cabbage into a blender or, if you feel it more appropriate, pound with a pestle and mortar. Squeeze the juice out through a muslin cloth and measure it. For each 600ml(1 pint) take 300ml(½ pint) of clear honey. Put the juice and honey into a heavy-bottomed pan and cook over a low heat, skimming when necessary, until the mixture is the consistency of syrup. When cold, bottle and seal. Take 1 teaspoon as needed for a persistent cough or 1 tablespoon a day as a precaution against catarrhal infection.

• *Cabbage or leek water* One of the most effective and nauseating-sounding cures for persistent catarrhal infections, which may cause both coughs and bronchitis, is the drinking of the warm water into which all the goodness of the cabbage or leeks has leeched during

cooking. Nasty though it sounds, it does taste quite savoury and should be taken night and morning. It is also an ancient remedy for whooping cough.

• *Pickled red cabbage* Eaten with its vinegar and mixed with honey this will also reduce a tickly cough.

• *Elecampane* Smelling deliciously of sultry violets, this is one of the oldest herbal remedies known to man for curing asthmatic conditions, and because it is a soothing bactericide it will clear painful respiratory problems.

Elecampane Honey
1 cup elecampane root
1 cup clear clover honey
1 cup water

Put all the ingredients into a stainless steel pan and bring gently to the boil. Reduce the heat and simmer until the root is soft. Strain and bottle.

Sweet Soothers, Shrubs and Cordials

Shrubs, robs, cordials and vinegars are marvellously old-fashioned antidotes to the common cough and cold and should be taken at the first sign of shivers and a tickly throat. They can of course be taken by the whole family at the onset of winter to prevent infections but fruit shrubs are not suitable for children who, however, will love the syrupy smoothness of fruit robs and cordials and the fizzy zing of fruit vinegar in hot water.

Blackcurrants, raspberries and elderberries or even a mixture of these soft fruits can be used in the recipe which follows to make a delightful shrub. Robs or cordials can be made in exactly the same way but omitting the brandy. Dilute shrubs and robs in the proportions of half liquor to half boiling water and drink whilst tucked up in bed prior to sleeping or take neat, a small teaspoon at a time, for an irritating cough.

Blackberry Shrub
1kg(2¼lb) blackberries
1 tablespoon each allspice berries and whole cloves, crushed
piece each cinnamon stick and nutmeg
clear mild honey
brandy

Place the blackberries in a pan with the crushed spices and just enough water to prevent sticking. Cover and simmer gently until soft then strain through a muslin cloth. Measure the resulting juice and for each 600ml(1 pint) have ready 200ml(7 fl oz) of honey and 150ml(¼ pint) of brandy. Return the juice and honey to a clean pan and stir over a low heat until the honey has dissolved. Bring to the boil then simmer for 10 minutes. Remove the pan from the heat and stir in the brandy. Bottle when cool. Seal with plastic-lined screw-top lids or corks. Store in a cool dark place.

● *Elderberry juice* The juice of elderberries has long been used to ease coughs, colds and sore throats whilst the juice or jelly of elderberries and/or blackcurrants was used to cure quinsy in children. Simmer 100g(4oz) of elderberries and 6 cloves in enough water to cover. When soft press them well into a sieve to extract all the juice. Sweeten with honey and drink hot 3 wineglasses full daily. Hot elderberry wine is wonderfully warming and soothing and so is hot elderberry rob.
● *Fruit vinegars* Raspberry vinegar can be made using frozen raspberries when fresh are unavailable and is as

useful in the kitchen as in the medicine cabinet. Many recipes suggest the inclusion of cinnamon and cloves, spices which have strong antiseptic qualities, but I find that their flavour overwhelms the delicacy of raspberries. If the vinegar is made with a more robust fruit such as blackcurrant, blackberry or elderberry then it is worth experimenting for the addition of spices is certainly beneficial. For a drink, dilute in the proportions of half vinegar, half hot water. This is particularly useful in soothing the kind of tickly cough that children find so distressing.

Raspberry Vinegar
1kg(2¼lb) raspberries
1 litre(1¾ pints) white malt vinegar
clear honey

Place the clean and carefully examined fruit in an earthenware or glass crock with the vinegar. Cover and leave for five days, stirring occasionally. Strain through a fine sieve or muslin then measure the juice gained and for each 600ml(1 pint) take 300ml(½ pint) honey. Put the juice or honey into a stainless steel or enamel pan and heat gently, stirring well. Bring to the boil then simmer for 10 minutes. Pour into warm dry bottles and seal with non-metal (plastic-lined) lids. Avoid metal because it becomes corroded by the vinegar which not only makes it impossible to reach the contents but also looks dangerously unappealing.

● *Blackcurrants* As well as all the delicious recipes given prior to this, a tablespoon of blackcurrant jam in a cup of very hot water is a good emergency standby to stop a night-time cough. Hot blackcurrant juice also relieves bronchial coughs whilst having the additional advantage of providing extra vitamin C.

● *Walnuts* The vinegar from preserved (pickled) walnuts mixed with honey will cure a night-time cough.

● *Liquorice and honey* As children we chewed liquorice root which had been dipped in clear honey to ease the type of persistent cough and sore throat that went with a full-blooded cold and it is an old-fashioned remedy that children do like. Once the piece of root has been chewed and sucked it should be thrown away before it begins to shred. The pleasure is in sucking all the flavour from it but it is not suitable for very small children. Instead a drink made from soaking a liquorice root in hot water until soft and then sweetening with honey can be given by the glass when needed. Although no longer sold in sweet shops liquorice root can still be bought in herbalists and wholefood shops.

● *Barley sugar* Sucking barley sugar sweets helps ease a sore throat basically by increasing salivation which is also why it stops children feeling car sick.

● *Eucalyptus oil B.P.* Three drops of eucalyptus oil on a sugar lump will stop coughing at night.

Herbal Teas, Drinks and Gargles

● *Thyme tea* Take 2 sprigs of the flowering tips of this fragrant herb and cover with 1 cup of boiling water. Take three times daily. Thyme is a powerful antiseptic. Hyssop tea can be made in the same way and will prove invaluable in easing a bronchial cough.

● *Elderflower or yarrow tea* Both are healing and calming.

● *Mullein tea* One teaspoon of mullein to 1 cup of boiling water taken three times a day will ease all types of coughs but especially the night-time tickles. The petals of mullein contain at least 10 per cent glucose and so have a pleasant enough taste to need no further sweetening.

● *Lungwort* Put in a pan in the proportions of 25g(1oz) to 600ml(1 pint) of water. Bring slowly to the boil and boil for three minutes. Remove from the heat, cover and infuse for 10 minutes. Strain and take three cups a day with or without honey. Lungwort, as the name signifies, works very well on chesty coughs.

● *Elecampane, coltsfoot, elderflower and horehound* Take 25g(1oz) each of these sedative, soothing and expectorant herbs, mix well and add to 1.1 litres(2 pints) of boiling water. Reduce to 600ml(1 pint) by simmering in a stainless steel or enamel pan. Leave to cool then stir in ½ teaspoon of cinnamon or cayenne. Drink 1 wineglass well sweetened with honey every three hours.

● *White horehound and marsh mallow infusion* Mix together an equal quantity of each herb and take 1 teaspoon at a time to 1 cup of boiling water. Sweeten with honey if liked and take three times daily. Marsh mallow is used in many remedies for bronchial complaints and is gentle enough for children to take.

● *Coltsfoot* The Latin name for this ancient herb which is still pictorially displayed in many pharmacies in Europe is *Tussilago Farfara* which may ring a bell with many mothers who have bought commercial cough linctus. It was undoubtedly recognized as a magic herb in the fight against catarrhal coughs and colds because of its high vitamin C content. It is necessary to strain the tea through a very close muslin as the downy leaves are covered in fine hairs which if swallowed are irritant. Leave 25g(1oz) of the dried leaves or flowers to soak in 600ml(1 pint) of cold water. Transfer to a stainless steel or enamel pan and bring gently to the boil. Remove from the heat, cover and infuse for 10 minutes. Strain through several layers of cloth and drink 4 cups a day with or without honey to ease all types of coughs. Coltsfoot rock or candy can still be bought from herbalists. It is very effective and children love it.

● *Eucalyptus for wheezy coughs* Many brand-name herbal remedies for coughs and colds contain soothing, antiseptic oil from the 'fever tree'. The following tea is very easy to make and is probably the most effective of all to ease a wheezy cough: boil 25g(1oz) of eucalyptus leaves in 600ml(1 pint) of water for 1 minute. Remove from the heat, cover and infuse for 10 minutes. Drink warm, 4 cups daily. It is also invaluable as a hot-water inhalant and eucalyptus leaves kept simmering in a small bowl of water in a sick room act as an antiseptic humidifier.

● *Eucalyptus for bronchial patients* Make a tea by infusing 5 eucalyptus leaves and 6 cloves in boiling water for five minutes and drink with lemon juice and honey. Several drops of oil of eucalyptus dropped into boiling water and used as an inhalant will bring relief from a bronchial cough. Always remember to keep warm after inhaling.

● *Honeysuckle* A fairy remedy that Christina Rossetti would have been proud of suggests that a child should sip the honeydew from the honeysuckle flower to stop a cough. Happily it is safe and really does work for very small children with very small coughs. More pragmatically and barbarously it is much more effective to infuse 15g(½oz) of honeysuckle blossoms in 1 litre(1¾ pints) of boiling water for 10 minutes. Peach blossoms also come in for equally

cavalier treatment: 3g(⅛oz) each of peach blossoms and honeysuckle blossoms to 1 cup of boiling water is a soothing, scented tea that will bring great pleasure to small children, particularly little girls.

● *Salt, lemon juice or cider vinegar* Any of these diluted in warm water make a safe antiseptic gargle to ease a tickling throat. Cider vinegar or lemon juice taken with honey and hot water will ensure a good night's sleep.

● *Sage gargle* Steep 25g(1oz) sage and a good pinch of cayenne pepper in 600ml(1 pint) of boiling water in a china tea pot for 12 hours to create a powerful gargle which will heal and refresh.

BRONCHITIS

Bronchitis is the step further that coughs and colds may well descend to if they have not been properly treated in the first place. The symptoms are an aching throat, tight chest, cough, headache and probably a temperature. Although it is an unpleasant ailment it should clear up within a few days but if it does not take professional advice. Most people suffering from bronchitis prefer to stay in bed, although in modern centrally heated houses this is no longer essential unless the illness is severe. Nevertheless it is sensible to ensure that the patient stays put in one heated room and does not wander into a cold kitchen or corridor. Make sure that children keep their chests well covered and their warm slippers on. Keeping a small pan of herbal water simmering in the room will act as a humidifier, keeping the air sweet and healthy. It is also important that the room is fresh and aired.

Fortunately most people will not suffer from bronchitis more than once in several years, if at all, and in most cases it is not a prolonged illness. Although it is rare today for bronchitis to linger over the years, in earlier times it was the rule rather than the exception and our forefathers took preventative steps at the beginning of each winter to ensure their continued good health. A piece of fat bacon – a substantial portion of pig rather than a slice of supermarket streaky – would be strapped to the chest beneath a permanent vest. Alternatively that vest might have been a garment of brown paper well impregnated with goose grease. In either case it would have been a barrier against catching a chest cold and have been considered 'wearable until unbearable'! Goose grease, presumably because of its availability (a good fat goose killed in the late autumn would have provided plenty of grease for several months) and the ease with which it is absorbed into the skin, was useful in medicinal rubs for the chest and the soles of the feet to protect them against rising damp. If one did succumb to illness a rigorous regime of hot mustard or kaolin poultices applied to the chest ensued or in extreme cases the wax from burning tallow candles was dripped on to brown paper and pressed on whilst still warm. The sight of all those candles burning must have given the victim cause for anxious thought.

Mustard foot baths were also used to comfort the sufferer. These had a double benefit of not only warming the body right through but also creating a warmly moist atmosphere in which to be cosseted. The ideal, of course, would be to have taken the foot bath whilst sitting before a roaring fire, a warm blanket around the shoulders, a fortifying toddy close at hand and, to ward off further infection, a string of onions garlanding one's head.

As children, when we suffered from wheezy colds my mother would rub our chests with a proprietary brand of camphorated liniment and although it brought considerable relief it had its drawbacks because the film of wax left upon the skin quickly became cold. To prevent this occurring we were kept in bed clutching well-covered hot-water bottles to our chests and fortified with hot lemon and honey or in extreme cases an aspirin.

Soothing Oils and Liniments

Friends of ours who make a regular pilgrimage to this country from the South of France to celebrate Christmas come armed in readiness for '*la Grippe*' with small bottles of aromatic oils with which they anoint themselves at every hour of day and night thus making their company an olfactory sensation. There are several similar recipes and they all come from either Southern Europe or Asia. They are used as everything from a chest rub to a liniment for sprained limbs. Many of the oils and liniments given under **Aches and Pains** are very effective in easing a wheezy cough and tight chest, particularly those which contain essential oils of eucalyptus, wintergreen, menthol, peppermint, hyssop, thyme, pine and oregano. Remember that they are more effective if applied warm to chest and throat and that the patient must keep his or her chest well covered afterwards. You could make up your own special favourite from any of the oils mentioned above or use a proprietary brand. A very easy liniment to make in an emergency is a few drops of camphor oil in 1 tablespoon of warm olive or sunflower oil. Oil-based liniments are preferable to those that are wax based as oil is more easily absorbed and does not leave a cold film on the skin.

● *Athena's oil* To ¼ cup of olive or sunflower oil add one drop each of the following warming and antiseptic essential oils: eucalyptus, pine, cinnamon, clove. Mix together and bottle. Use to relieve congestion by massaging it into the afflicted area of nose, sinus (taking care to avoid the eyes), throat and chest. A few drops of oil on pillow or handkerchief will help children breathe more easily and if sprinkled on a handkerchief and taken to school or work will create an effective barrier against other people's infections. The same oil can also be used as an inhalant in the quantities of 1 coffee spoon to 1 litre(1¾ pints) of boiling water.

● *Garlic* It would be very hard to find any ailment that garlic does not come to the aid of. Chop 6 cloves of garlic very finely and place them in a bowl over a pan of simmering water with the contents of one small jar of white petroleum jelly (vaseline). Cover and leave to simmer gently for several hours. Repot and use warm to rub into the back and chest. To be doubly effective the old wives might well have advocated that burdock leaves should be placed, furry sides down, between the shoulder blades at the same time.

Cough Mixtures

Most of the mixtures and syrups given under **Coughs** and some of those suggested to soothe **Asthma** and **Hayfever** will work very well on bronchial patients. However there are a few more which are specifically expectorant and soothing.

Hyssop Syrup
450g(1lb) clear honey
50g(2oz) fresh or 25g(1oz) dried hyssop
1 teaspoon crushed aniseed
1 piece crushed liquorice root
1 piece crushed root ginger

Put the honey into a stainless steel pan and heat gently to boiling point, skimming as you go. Add the remaining ingredients, stir well, cover and simmer gently for 30 minutes by which time the honey should taste quite strongly of hyssop. Strain and pour into hot, dry jars. Seal when cold. The syrup can be added to hot herbal teas or taken by the teaspoon when necessary.

● *Carrot juice* Drunk hot this will ease bronchitis and improve upon the general state of health.

● *Lemon in wine* Take the grated zest of ½ a well-washed lemon and macerate in a glass of hot wine with a spoonful of honey. Taken three times a day this not surprisingly promotes sweating and is quite relaxing!

● *Slippery elm* Mix the powdered bark to a palatable drinking consistency with warm water and honey and season with a good pinch of cayenne. Take morning and night. This is preferable to the ancient remedy of blackthorn bark peeled from the bush and boiled in water and sugar.

Inhalants

There are many useful inhalants mentioned under **Coughs**, **Asthma**, **Hayfever** and **Colds**, the most popular of which are eucalyptus and Friar's balsam (tincture of benzoin). Any of the essential oils mentioned under Soothing Oils and Liniments for bronchitis can be used a few drops at a time in hot water and inhaled or to impregnate a handkerchief.

● *Essential oil of juniper* A few drops may be used in hot water as an inhalant. Do not use undiluted on the skin or on a handkerchief where it will be transferred to the nose.
● *Garlic* Several cut cloves of garlic in a bowl of boiling water make an unusual but effective inhalant.
● *Coltsfoot* A tobacco made from this herb was used to relieve bronchitis and asthma but it is in your best interests not to smoke at all.

Diet

Eat plenty of fresh, juicy fruit and fresh green vegetables. Pineapples and grapes were considered particularly beneficial to the health of invalids but as in times past the average family would have found them very difficult to obtain this may well have brought them into the realms of emotional blackmail. Take plenty of fluids but avoid milk if catarrh is present. Both onions and garlic, chewed raw, were thought to speed recovery but I suspect that this was one way to ensure that everybody gave the patient a wide berth thus reducing the risk of spreading the infection!

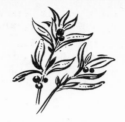

PNEUMONIA

The warnings that accompany old-fashioned treatments for pneumonia or 'congestion of the lungs' were so dire that even as late as the 1930s almost no hope was given out for the patient's recovery and I can find no remedy which was put forward in the genuine belief that it would succeed. Although matters are vastly improved today there is no doubt that if you or a member of your family suffer from a bad cough, pains in the chest and a high temperature, particularly when influenza is rife, you should immediately seek professional advice. This is especially relevant if the victim is very young or elderly, is not of a normally healthy constitution or is just recovering from a previous illness.

If the infection is not of the most serious kind any of the remedies given in this section will be useful. Patients convalescing from a more serious illness will also gain relief and strength from these recipes. People who are very ill rarely want to eat but it is important that they drink plenty. Keep the room well aired and keep a small bowl of eucalyptus or lavender simmering in order to promote a pleasant atmosphere. An old-fashioned idea for keeping the patient comfortable is to bathe the face with warm water into which 1 tablespoon of cider or lavender vinegar has been stirred then wipe dry with paper tissues which should afterwards be burned. Other ideas for nursing feverish patients can be found under **Colds, Sneezing and Influenza**.

● *Honey and lemon* One dessertspoon of honey to the juice of ½ lemon to be taken every half hour.
● *Slippery elm* Mix 3 dessertspoons of the powdered bark to a drinkable consistency with water, add honey to sweeten and take twice daily at six-hourly intervals.
● *Cinnamon and lemon juice* Add the juice of ½ a lemon and ¼ teaspoon of cinnamon to a coffee cup of boiling water. Allow to cool. Gargle with the mixture to relieve a sore throat and then swallow. Avoid this remedy, however, if you suffer from heartburn.
● *A healing tea* Take 25g(1oz) of each of the following herbs: agrimony, salad burnet, meadowsweet, wood betony, raspberry leaves (best avoided if you are pregnant). Mix the herbs and add them to 1 litre(1¾ pints) of boiling water. Simmer for 20 minutes and when cool season with cinnamon and a few drops of lemon juice. Administer 1 wineglass every hour.

PLEURISY

This is a particularly uncomfortable and, for children, frightening illness which affects the lung or lungs and which, again, has been given a wide berth in the records of folk medicine as a result, I suspect, of the poor recovery rate amongst its victims. Although requiring professional attendance pleurisy is no longer considered quite so dangerous. The first signs are of chill and shivers accompanied by a dry cough and a sharp pain in the side when coughing or sneezing or moving suddenly. Those who were particularly vulnerable were the young and elderly and those who had been exposed to severe cold and damp or who had been suffering from infections relating to the chest. To add to the anxiety pleurisy was often considered to be the first sign of consumption so a careful wife and mother made sure that her family were adequately clothed to protect them against such an eventuality. Strong warnings were issued never to remove underclothing from the chest in winter, to keep red flannel next to the skin and that children should be dressed beneath the bedclothes in cold weather. Even as late as the mid 20th century baths were advised against in houses that did not have heating. The mothers of Britain were advised to administer to their infants 'a good wash of the face, hands and private parts, avoiding exposure to draughts and chill as a little honest dirt must be much preferred to the consequence of illness'.

When you consider the treatments recommended for pleurisy the consequences of this illness were indeed unpleasant: saline purgatives and diuretics to remove liquid from the lungs, blistering to draw excess liquid through the skin or a heavy strapping of plaster from backbone to breastbone to prevent movement and relieve pain – that is until the moment of removal which, if you were a hairy-chested fellow, must have made the eyes water.

Poultices of boiled nettles, lungwort or linseed meal were all recommended as was the same green poultice using cabbage that is given for **Cramp** and I am quite certain that any of these gentle country poultices, used warm, would have brought about a certain amount of welcome relief from pain.

The best advice, however, is to send the patient to bed. Do not force them to lie down if to do so causes them pain or impairs their breathing. Make sure that they are nice and warm, especially their feet, and that the room is warm but well aired. Encourage them to take plenty of fluids, especially those that will promote a gentle perspiration and those that will aid healing.

Many of the recipes given under **Bronchitis** and **Coughs** will bring relief and so will the suggestions for soothing applications of warm herbal oil (see page 4) gently massaged into the painful side of the chest. Make sure that plenty of fresh fruit and vegetables are eaten and avoid allowing the patient to become constipated as this will make them feel considerably worse.

Well-Tried Remedies

● *Toastwater* Good home-made bread, dried in the oven to a powder and boiled in water with butter and salt is the best and most old-fashioned drink to take in cases of pleurisy and pneumonia.
● *Bran tea* Boil 1 good tablespoon of bran in 1 litre(1¾ pints) of water. Skim and leave to stand for a few minutes then strain and add a large spoonful of honey. Drink hot during the day.

● *Black molasses* Take 1 dessertspoon every three hours for the first day reducing to every six hours for the succeeding days of illness.
● *Pleurisy root or butterfly weed* A tea made from the root of the North American plant *Asclepias tuberosa* was one of the only cures for pleurisy available to the early settlers in America. The active principle of the root, asclepin, is still used as a fluid extract in commercial medicines.

A Herbal Tea to Relieve Pleurisy
15g(½oz) cayenne
50g(2oz) raspberry leaves
50g(2oz) yarrow
1¾ litres(3 pints) boiling water

Mix the cayenne and herbs together and add them to the water. Boil for 30 minutes and drink 1 glass of the cool liquid every two hours. Do not use this tea if the patient is pregnant.

● *Elderflower tea, hyssop tea, hyssop syrup, cabbage leaf poultice or daisy infusion (wine)* These will all stave off incipient pleurisy when other chest infection is present.

Colds, Sneezing and Influenza

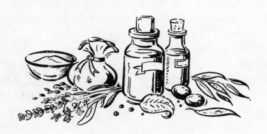

'Atishoo, atishoo, we all fall down.' In this terrifying parody of the effects of the plague sneezing was shown to be one of the first symptoms. Modern theorists now believe that many of these deadly epidemics were devastasting forms of influenza which, because people were less well equipped both physically and medically to cope with it, carried off great numbers, particularly children and the elderly, to an untimely death.

To our forefathers, however, even the common cold represented a dire threat for, unable to place their reliance upon a miracle cure from the National Health Service and without sickness benefit to sustain them, a heavy cold meant at best an unpaid absence from work or at worst serious and prolonged illness which could become complicated and lead ultimately to death. Without the benefits, doubtful or otherwise, of central heating, air conditioning and easily available covered transport our great-grandmothers took care to see that adequate precautions were taken with correct and sufficient clothing and fuel food to sustain the body under the most adverse conditions. Care was essential to prevent the worst from happening but if it did a mustard bath, a hot drink and plenty of warm covering administered with a swift prayer to the Almighty to be merciful were the only immediate solutions.

Care took the form of year-round vigilance combined with the inherited wisdom of knowing and understanding what would ensure continued good health: which fruits to put by for winter use, the barrels of apples stored for daily consumption, the berries and soft fruit full of valuable vitamins, the flowers and leaves with antiseptic and healing qualities which could be drunk, sucked or burned when illness stalked the countryside. Prevention, although not easy, was infinitely better than having to cure.

Apart from ensuring 'an apple a day' and a daily intake of fresh fruit and vegetables, how else might we guard against the common cold? The suggestions from time immemorial varied vastly, ranging from dried swallow's bones wrapped in vine leaves and carried around the neck (presumably if you were in a position to obtain anything quite so esoteric you were also in a position to follow the live swallow abroad and avoid winter cold) to honeysuckle syrup.

Garlic, a clove a day, has a justifiable reputation as being a remarkable cold preventative and cure. If you object to the taste and smell, perles and capsules are equally effective and less offensive. I suspect that apart from having extremely potent antiseptic qualities, the chewing of garlic is so antisocial that no one comes close enough to transmit their own germs. If you do not suffer from catarrh, drinking milk in which 2 garlic cloves have been boiled is to be recommended as effective and less pungent. I am constantly amazed that garlic enjoys such a reputation as an aphrodisiac. Presumably the therapeutic qualities of the herb are so stimulating that the libido is provoked to the point where all else can be ignored. My own particular preference for garlic is in salad dressing and I find that when the body is exhausted and at its lowest ebb the finest and most restorative meal that one can enjoy is hot crusty garlic bread accompanying a large bowl of home-made onion soup.

In what other ways might the conscientious wife and mother protect her family against taking a chill? There are within the pages of a good housewife's manual methods of prevention which would have interested the Spanish Inquisition, ranging from sewing the family into flannel at the end of Septem-ber and releasing them in May, after which 'the casting of the clout' must have required nerves of steel and a strong stomach, to an evil-sounding mustard poultice applied hot upon the chest which would have been so fraught with hazard as to make it impractical.

A last word from the medical profession upon prescribing for the common cold: 'If I prescribe for a patient a cold will be cleared up within seven days and if I do not it will hang around for about a week.'

Hot Possets

These hot and comforting drinks will warm a cold body and stimulate the circulation thus warding off the dangers of 'taking a chill'.

Grandad Fred's Hot Toddy Mixture
1 piece root ginger
2 teaspoons caraway seed
1 bottle whisky
grated zest and juice of 1 lemon
350g(12oz) light muscovado sugar
225g(8oz) raisins (large, fat, sticky variety)

Bruise the ginger and caraway seeds and put them into a wide-necked jar with all the other ingredients. Seal tightly and leave for three weeks, shaking daily, then strain and re-bottle. Drunk by itself or with hot water this toddy is said to cure everything from an incipient cold to sea sickness but it is to be recommended only as a deterrent because too much alcohol taken when the body is fighting a fever burns up valuable vitamin C.

• *Honey and lemon* Once again and in a variety of different ways this famous and already well-recommended cure-all will alleviate the symptoms of a cold and also comfort when misery takes over. Drink it hot and undiluted or with hot water and flavour with cinnamon, cloves, ginger or cayenne or even a mixture of each or some of these. It is also excellent with whisky, brandy or ginger cordial. A very good alcoholic ginger cordial can be made by using the above 'Grandad Fred's' recipe but substituting brandy for the whisky and using a more substantial chunk of root ginger.

● *Gingered beer* Ginger mulled in beer is an old-fashioned remedy which improves sleep and is especially useful for restless fellows.

● *Honey and eucalyptus* Mix 1 teaspoon of honey into a small coffee cup of hot water and add 3 drops of essential oil of eucalyptus. Take two or three times a day. Eucalyptus is also first rate when used as an inhalant in hot water.

● *Hot milky drinks* These are excellent when children or adults alike are cold, wet and tired and they usually ensure a sound night's sleep. However milk may aggravate catarrhal conditions. Although I do not advocate trying the old Asian favourite of hot yak milk, grated garlic and ghee there are plenty of other soothing ideas which certainly help small children feel cosseted and comforted, thus winning half the battle, especially if it helps them to sleep without distress. Freshly ground cinnamon or ginger stirred into hot milk is antiseptic and warming but do not boil the milk as this destroys much of its goodness. Hot chocolate sweetened with honey can be substituted for the milk: popped into a blender to give it a frothy head and decorated with one of the previously mentioned spices and a smattering of grated chocolate it will look too good for even the tetchiest child to pass up.

● *Hot milk and onion* A large sliced onion simmered in milk is as good for you as onion soup. Some people suggest tripe and onions made with milk while others substitute garlic for the onions. If you do not like milk simmer your onions in water. Many remedies advocate seasoning with cayenne.

● *Cayenne* Half a teaspoon of cayenne pepper added to 150ml($\frac{1}{4}$ pint) of hot milk or water is very warming but it is not appreciated by children. Do make sure that the pepper is well dissolved otherwise it may be a little more warming than intended.

● *Bread and milk* Butter slices of bread and sprinkle them with sugar. Cover with hot milk and eat before going to bed. This delicious 'milk mess' will send you to sleep without a qualm when you are tired and cold.

Cold Comfort

One of the first signs of illness is an excessive thirst which becomes worse as the body burns up energy combating infection, and which has the patient demanding coffee, tea and fizzy drinks, none of which are particularly good for them. A century ago none of these would have been easily or economically available and bran or barley waters and herb tea were used, not only to reduce thirst but to prevent dehydration and alleviate the problem with their own healing properties.

Lemon Barley Water
1 large lemon
2 tablespoons pearl barley
1 litre(1$\frac{3}{4}$ pints) boiling water

Pare the rind thinly from the well-washed lemon and place it with the barley in a large heatproof jug. Pour on the boiling water, cover and leave to stand overnight. The next day strain off the pale straw-coloured liquid and drink by the glass with or without honey. Save the juice from the lemons to make another drink but do not add it to the barley water. This is an inexpensive drink which soothes and nourishes and should be made fresh daily.

Lemonade
2 lemons
1 litre(1¾ pints) water
50g(2oz) sugar

Wash the lemon well and remove the rind using a potato peeler, taking care not to include any of the white pith. Put the rind into a pan with half the water and the sugar and bring gently to the boil, stirring well to make sure the sugar has dissolved. Cover and simmer for a few minutes. Pour into a jug and leave to get cold. Strain then add the juice from the lemons and the remaining water. Serve as it is.

Ginger Lemon Cordial
6 lemons
4 oranges
150g(4oz) seedless raisins
3 cups clear honey
75g(3oz) ginger root, crushed
4.5 litres(8 pints) water

Wash the lemons and oranges well then grate the rind from them and squeeze the juice, which should be kept in the refrigerator until needed. Put the rinds and remaining ingredients into a large pan and bring to the boil. Simmer for one hour. Skim and leave in jugs overnight to cool. Add the fruit juices the next day. Drink undiluted.

● *Apple tea* Slice washed but unpeeled apples and place them in a saucepan with just enough water to cover. Simmer for one hour, strain and use hot or cold. This health-giving drink cuts colds to the quick. With honey added and diluted with sparkling mineral water it also makes a very good summertime drink.

● *Fruit juices* Any fruit juice that has a good sharp flavour and contains vitamin C must improve one's state of health at the same time as it is refreshing the beleaguered body. Blackcurrant, loganberry, apple, pineapple, lemon and orange all spring instantly to mind although it is now suggested that people who constantly suffer from catarrhal infection should avoid orange juice as it is believed to exacerbate the condition. Both grape juice and pomegranate juice are wonderfully thirst-quenching and apart from being of physical value it is also thought that they bring peace of mind and promote pure thoughts! Grated, dried pomegranate peel soaked in a small cup of boiling water then strained makes an excellent gargle for sore throats. Children who are feeling unwell with a rotten cold will relish eating the raw pomegranate, seed by delicious crystal seed, which will also do them a lot of good. Although all of these fruit juices will cool the patient down, and for that reason give them instant relief, many people believe that it is more rewarding to take all fruit juices hot with honey.

Refreshing Herbal Teas

All herbal teas are soothing and are taken to promote healing and those teas which make the traditional reviving breakfast cuppa are also herbs whether they come from India, China or Ceylon. Taken with honey and lemon they will refresh and stimulate. The following herb teas are those which are more suitable to remedy colds, flu and catarrhal infections.

• *Yarrow and horehound tea* This has the dual and doubtful role as both a classic cold and cough cure and an unparalleled love philtre, probably based on the premise that the light of one's life would only respond to romantic overtures when one was in the peak of condition which, in the days of our forefathers, may not have been too often.

• *Camomile, elder and lime flower tea* The flowers mixed in equal proportion make an excellent, delicately flavoured floral tea which children love and which also induces a gentle perspiration. To give relief to a troublesome night-time tickle make the tea with an infusion of liquorice root and honey water which should be strained and brought to the boil again before pouring over the herbs.

• *Elderflower, peppermint leaf and yarrow tea* Mixed in equal quantities and combined with a pinch of mixed spice these provide a tea which not only promotes perspiration but also acts as a mild digestive, settling the type of queasy stomach so often attendant upon fever and catarrh. Both elderflower and peppermint tea and elderberry and peppermint tea are almost equally effective and will also ease a tickly cough if taken with honey and lemon. Failing either, a few drops of essential oil of peppermint or a tablespoon of peppermint cordial in hot water are very soothing.

• *Angelica tea* This or a few drops of essential oil of angelica in a cup of hot water will clear a stuffy nose and improve the sense of smell. It can also be inhaled. Angelica and nettle tea fortifies and soothes.

• *Other herbal tea mixtures* All the following have been well tried and tested to bring proven relief: sage or sage and grapefruit zest; borage, agrimony and hyssop in equal quantities; fenugreek; camomile; coltsfoot; rose petal and rose hip tea (obtained commercially); self-heal or self-heal and alkanet.

• *Basil tea* Made with either fresh or dried leaves basil tea brings about a mild perspiration and with the addition of a pinch of ground cloves and cinnamon not only reduces fever but has a perfume so heady and redolent of hot Mediterranean heaths that it invokes a dreamy calm.

• *Spice tea* Take 1 stick of cinnamon, 2 cloves and 2 sprigs of fresh or 3 pinches of dried thyme and boil gently in 1 litre(1¾ pints) of water for two minutes. Infuse for three minutes before straining and drinking.

• *Tamarind tea* Take 1 cup of tamarind pulp to 1 litre(1¾ pints) of boiling water. Cover and leave to infuse for two hours. Strain and drink, ½ a cup at a time and sweetened with a little honey, every four hours.

• *Ginger tea* Infuse a good chunk of bruised fresh ginger root in hot water or chew on a small piece. If masochism is not part of your make-up sprinkle ¼ teaspoon of ground ginger into a cup of hot water and add 2 teaspoons of honey to make a pleasant drink.

Soothing Wines, Syrups and Mixtures

Most old-fashioned and herbal syrupy concoctions which are given to relieve the misery of colds and coughs have several benefits. Many of them contain ingredients which encourage the body to resist infection, others promote perspiration – the belief being that this helps to rid the system of fever more rapidly – whilst others again soothe sore and tickly throats and relieve congested noses and sinuses. All of these are preferable to drugs which 'dry up' a cold and which frequently leave the patient with inflamed and sensitive mucous membranes, cracked lips and a parched feeling both externally and internally.

Hot blackcurrant syrup and rose hip syrup are already well established in this country as methods of preventing colds from occurring in children whilst in South America the fruit of the acerola cherry (*Malfigia funicifolia*) is stewed with honey to provide a health-giving syrup. The fruit is, in fact, so high in vitamin C that it is exported in quantity to North America to make health drinks for children. The French also use a sharp, red cherry to make a syrup which is given to relieve the symptoms of a cold, whilst Middle Eastern people stew figs gently in a syrup of lemon and honey to achieve the same delicious result. We already know that hot lemon and honey relieves all the most unpleasant effects of a cold but a spoonful of molasses taken in hot water is also extremely beneficial, although I feel that one might draw the line at mullein pounded in molasses which, although it does you good, tastes revolting. Another very useful prevent-ative if taken regularly, but equally dif-ficult to get down, is ¼ teaspoon of wheatgerm oil in honey. Perhaps it might be more palatable stirred into the morning cereal or yoghurt.

The British, however, were brought up on cod liver oil and malt and we must be grateful that we did not live a century or so ago when brimstone and treacle or a mixture of sugar, butter and vinegar might have been forced down our unwilling throats. In even more typically stoical British fashion both rowan berries and elderberries were made into a strong, astringent syrup to cure the common cold. These fruits were considered so beneficial that

travellers abroad would often take a pocketful of the dried berries with them to guard against infection and history has it that this was how the blueberry found its way to North America.

Coltsfoot Syrup
50g(2oz) fresh coltsfoot leaves
1 litre(1¾ pints) water
8 tablespoons clear honey

Make sure that your freshly picked leaves are clean and free from any creepy crawlies. Wash well, drain and place in a large stainless steel or enamel pan with the water. Bring to the boil, skim, cover and simmer gently for 30 minutes. Leave to cool for a few minutes then strain into a clean pan. Add the honey and heat gently, stirring continuously until it has melted, then boil steadily for 10 minutes without covering. Skim once again and strain through a fine nylon mesh. Leave until quite cold before pouring into small bottles. Seal and keep refrigerated. Take 1 tablespoon every four hours for a cough and cold. It has a lovely fresh flavour and children like it very much. Provided you have made it correctly and kept it in the refrigerator it should last well too.

● *White turnip syrup* Take a large, white turnip, wash it well and shave the bottom until it is flat. Cut it in half and divide each piece into four slices. Spread each piece thickly on both sides with honey and place them all back together again to make a whole. Stand this in a close-fitting china bowl and trickle 2 tablespoons of honey over the top. Cover with a cloth and leave over-night. Drink the syrup that collects in the bottom of the bowl, 1 teaspoon at a time, for the type of tickly cough that goes with a cold. I have to mention that this recipe was given to me by a reader from abroad who assured me that not only did it work but it also did not taste as nasty as it sounds. She was quite right on both counts, but do call it by another name when offering it to the patient.

● *Elderberry wine* Taken hot at night it is a marvellous antidote to the snuffles. So is elderberry syrup.

Elderberry Syrup
a good quantity of fresh elderberries
sugar or honey
whole cloves

Put the elderberries in a large fireproof dish and leave to stand overnight in a warm oven. Pour off the juice and put the fruit back in the oven. Repeat this until there is no more juice left, then give the fruit a quick squeeze in a muslin cloth to remove any last drops. Measure the juice and for each 1 litre(1¾ pints) take 450g(1lb) of sugar or honey and 12 cloves. Put all the ingredients in a large stainless steel or enamel pan and heat gently, stirring well until the sugar is dissolved, then simmer for 30 minutes. Skim, strain and bottle. Seal well and keep refrigerated. Drink as it is or diluted with hot water at bed time or when a cold awakes one from sleep. Do not use rowan berries in the same way as they are too astringent.

Trying Anything Once

The common cold has defeated scientists for centuries and, despite the money, intelligence and vast pharmaceutical resources poured into researching a cure, will probably continue to defeat us for years to come. Many of the strange and seemingly illogical folk methods of curing, or at least of allevi-

ating, the misery of colds have their basis in strong commonsense and a more than passing knowledge of anatomy. Many of them work surprisingly well and are frequently given an airing by research groups and clinics.

Some of us have found that splashing the face with cold water will relieve the misery of running eyes and nose and sneezes. Hayfever sufferers will have tried sea water, ice bags, sniffing copious snorts of water up each nostril and complete immersion daily. Since civilized man endowed the Eskimos with the common cold they have discovered their own method of curing it by sniffing snow up their noses and there is a very good reason for this and any other 'cold nose' cure. The icy cold snow contracts the swollen membranes within the nose and this in turn creates an expulsion of accumulated mucus The mucous membranes are no longer irritated and inflamed and the 'cold' disappears.

Without the help of ice and snow you can make your own remedy by taking 2 cups of ice-cold water (place the water in the freezing compartment of your refrigerator for a few minutes) and stirring into it 1 teaspoon of bicarbonate of soda and 1 tablespoon of Epsom salts. Stir well and then dip a folded cloth into the solution. Wring out the excess water and place the cloth over the nose and sinuses for as long as it takes for some relief to become apparent. Keep the solution cold and the cloth refreshed.

Other methods of trying to stop the nose streaming and to stop sneezing are to sniff sea water, warm water and lemon juice, neat lemon juice or sage vinegar. Rubbing a sage leaf around the nose was considered useful, probably because the natural oils in sage are antiseptic and healing, and it is certainly less painful than lemon juice or vinegar both of which work on the principle, I believe, of shrivelling the mucous membrane with shock. John Wesley was no less gentle in his approach to sneezing and advocated the coiled rind of a thinly pared orange up each nostril. Orris root was also used as a snuff and, although rather more pleasant than the alternative suggestion of cayenne, would have done nothing more than produce the most vigorous attack of sneezing, thus ridding the nasal passages of obstruction but hardly soothing and cooling. Most of the best methods suggested for easing sneezing either cool or lubricate these sensitive areas and do not rely upon 'drying up' a cold.

A very simple nasal spray which will ease the misery of early-morning sneezing is made by adding 1 teaspoon of fine sea salt and 2 tablespoons of glycerine to 2 cups of water (soft, bottled). Pour this into a sterilised jar and shake well. Use in an atomizer. I have been told that ladies would carry a small atomizer of eau de Cologne or lavender water in their handbags to use in an emergency.

Cold cures can also work beyond the easily acceptable fact of icy inhalation reaching into the realms of related pain. A friend of mine sits with his toes in a basin of freezing cold water. He had read that the Chinese believe that all areas of the body are directly associated and that freezing one's big toes causes the swollen membranes in nose, sinuses and throat to contract, which in turn reduces the irritation without harmful after-effects (although he does run the risk of frostbite). I have tried this suggestion and I have to say that it does appear to work but I would not have bowed to John Wesley's theory which insisted that not only toes but the whole body be subjected to an icy cold bath.

More conventional friends recommend 1 tablespoon each of mustard powder and household soda to a bucket of very warm water in which one immerses the feet whilst sitting with blankets wrapped around shoulders and waist. A hot-water bottle on the feet is another old-fashioned suggestion in direct contradiction to the frozen toe theory.

Food and sleep figure strongly and in a contradictory manner: do you feed a fever and starve a cold, or is it vice versa? Should we wrap up warmly and take a long, brisk walk? Or should we take the sensible advice of a writer on the subject of influenza who stated unequivocally, 'I cannot stress strongly enough the necessity for the patient to stay in bed for a long period of convalescence after this dangerous illness. To arise too soon and to attempt to carry out one's normal duties can, I fear, lead only to paralysis and insanity.' Strong words but bearing in mind the at present fashionable belief that M.E. (myalgic encephalomyelitis) may be the result of 'flu perhaps we should not scoff.

Delving into the realms of fantasy also provides some entertaining theories. Certain tribes of North American Indians chewed the leaf of the creosote bush to ward off colds whilst sailors of a century or so ago chewed tarred rope, both of which probably contained some of the constituents of modern-day medicines. Country folk slept with a piece of garlic or liquorice root between teeth and cheek or carried a piece of black sheep's wool well larded with butter or olive oil and egg around their necks. All of these remedies to keep infection away worked, I am sure, on the principle that you did not smell sufficiently pleasant to get close enough to infect although none could possibly be quite so effective as the Russian solution of tying a hank of dried herring around the throat. Centuries ago, when the threat of plague was close, anyone venturing out into the streets carried posies of strongly aromatic and anti-septic herbs to ward off infection. Within living memory small children were sent to school with a small purse of asafoetida or camphor tied beneath their collars, whilst in Mediterranean countries garlic was the chosen herb. All of these smelt equally pungent but were probably no worse than our latter-day preference for eucalyptus, winter-green and menthol.

Inhalants, Rubs and Gargles

The majority of the recipes and remedies to be found under **Chest Infections**, **Coughs** and **Asthma** work equally well on patients suffering from a cold or 'flu.

● *Friar's balsam* (tincture of benzoin) Inhaling the fumes of Friar's balsam was the acme of modern medicine in our home when I was a child.

● *Sage, peppermint, golden rod or basil leaves and elder, lime, camomile, lavender or verbascum flowers* One handful of fresh, or 1 tablespoon of dried, of any one or a mixture of these herbs in 1.5 litres (3 pints) of boiling water makes a gently effective and pleasing inhalant. Always remember to keep warm after inhaling.

● *Onions* Make a strong brew of onions, the steam of which should be inhaled through mouth and nose. It goes without saying that garlic is also recommended. A good strong sniff of raw onion was also believed to drive a cold away!

● *Olbas Oil* This may be used as a hot-water inhalant but is much better if applied to handkerchief or tissue.

(Always burn tissues, most especially when colds are in evidence.)

● *Essential oils of eucalyptus, thyme, camphor and cloves* Use these severally or together, adding a few drops to boiling water to make a soothing inhalant.

● *Eucalyptus, camomile or angelica rub* The essential oils of any of these, a few drops at a time, added to 1 tablespoon of almond or sunflower oil, can be used to gently massage the congested areas of face and throat. The two latter herbs are particularly kind and soothing on the sensitive areas around eyes and nose.

● *Gargles* Gargle with a few drops of iodine in a large glass of warm water. Quinine is reputed to have the same healing effect. A tea cup of barley water with 1 teaspoon each of salt and vinegar stirred in is also a reasonably gentle gargle.

Starve a Cold

It is undoubtedly better for a patient who is suffering from a bad cold or influenza to eat as little as possible and in fact they will probably reject most foods unreservedly. Staunchly old-fashioned remedies such as milk, but-ter, honey and garlic or onion, barley water and cod liver oil, which were designed to both prevent and cure colds, will do nothing to improve that situation. Onions are comforting and warming with many therapeutic quali-ties and so are garlic and many herbs, all of which can be incorporated into a nourishing broth. Beef tea and chicken soup were great favourites as was blancmange, particularly a savoury variety made with carragheen. Fruit sorbet made with orange or lemon juice or one of the soft fruits high in vitamin C slides down a sore throat without trouble whilst porridge is warm, sustaining, easily digested and a great improvement upon gruel. The best food, though, for sad and sorry people is yoghurt with wheatgerm and honey.

Fruit juices have already been mentioned and both grape juice and the juice of carrots are thought to improve the chances of a good recovery. Some sources have also been known to advocate the juice of turnip tops which are very good for you but perhaps better served up as a vegetable with a lemon and oil dressing. However there are plenty of very pleasant and appetising foods to choose from which will both tempt the patient to eat and also improve their general state of health. More importantly they are excellent nourishment to take when the body is cold and weary and at its most vulnerable.

Onion Soup
4 large onions
1 large clove garlic
5 tablespoons olive oil
¼ teaspoon each dried thyme, sage and savory
small piece of bay leaf
1 litre(1¾ pints) good strong chicken or vegetable stock
1 tablespoon fresh lemon juice
salt and freshly ground black pepper

Peel the onions and cut them into very thin slices and finely chop the garlic. Put the oil into a large saucepan and cook the onions and garlic in this until they are golden brown and transparent. Do not allow them to burn. Stir in the herbs and add the warmed stock a little at a time followed by the lemon juice, salt and pepper to taste. Cover and simmer very gently for one hour. Children will prefer the soup strained and it should be served hot with garlic and tomato bread (see below). I prefer to give invalids this onion soup rather than the thicker one made with milk which may exacerbate catarrhal infections. Truly strong men will take their soup liberally laced with cayenne pepper for maximum benefit.

● *Garlic and tomato bread* Bake thick slices of bread in a hot oven until lightly golden brown. Smear each side with a cut garlic clove, paste well with olive oil and spread with tomato purée.

Ghenghis Khan's Mustard
1 cup freshly grated horseradish
1 clove garlic
1 tablespoon sea salt
600ml(1 pint) boiling water
mustard powder and cayenne to taste

Mix the horseradish, garlic and salt together and cover with the boiling water. Leave to stand overnight in a china bowl. The next day strain then mix in the mustard powder and cayenne and beat until you have a thick paste. Pot in small jars and seal tightly when cold. Keep refrigerated. Whilst grating your fresh horseradish take care not to let the fumes get into your eyes nor to touch the sensitive areas of the face with your fingers otherwise you may end up with eyes and nose streaming more violently than that of your patient. This mustard can be used as an accompaniment to cold meat but spread on a slice of good bread and used to dunk in a soup it clears the head remarkably well, although it is not to be recommended for children.

● *Sweet suckets* During the prolific summer months fruits and often herbs were made into 'suckets' both to preserve them and to provide an easily acceptable source of valuable vitamins for children. Modern mothers will find that these pastilles and candies are a wonderfully healthy alternative to humbugs especially if their nearest and dearest travel on those great breeding grounds of the common cold and 'flu – the school bus and commuter train. Blackcurrants make the best pastilles because not only are they high in vitamin C but they also have a sharply delicious taste. Apples, blackberries and quince can be added to the choice of fruits which will enable you to keep the winter bugs at bay.

Blackcurrant Pastilles
1kg(2¼lb) blackcurrants
1 glass water
soft light brown sugar

Wash the currants and place them in a stainless steel pan (do not use aluminium, not only because of the recent discovery of a connection with Alzheimer's disease but because cooking in aluminium destroys valuable vitamin C) with the water, cover and simmer until quite soft. Pass through a fine sieve. Weigh the resulting purée and take its equivalent weight in sugar. Return the purée and sugar to a clean pan and cook gently, stirring continuously, until the mixture is thick enough to leave the sides of the pan with no excess moisture. Dust several shallow tins lightly with caster sugar and spread the paste reasonably thickly. Leave in a warm, dry place to harden enough to cut into small lozenges. This may take several days so do not panic and think that you have failed. Dust them with caster sugar and place in a cool oven to dry out completely. Store in airtight tins.

● *Angelica* Candied angelica stems can be chewed to counteract a sore throat and sniffles and also the loss of the sense of smell caused by heavy catarrh. Commercially produced crystallized angelica is expensive so try growing your own magnificently green and shady plant. Avoid taking angelica just before going to bed as it is a mild stimulant.

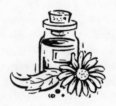

SINUSITIS

An unpleasantly painful ailment, sinusitis is the result of the mucous membrane linings of the sinus cavities around the eyes and leading to the nose becoming inflamed. The causes for this occurring are referred to under **Coughs** and **Catarrhal Infections** and the effects are very similar: a blocked-up feeling in the nose, slight temperature, tickly cough, headache and excruciating pain in and around those cavities particularly above the eyes. Many of the remedies, particularly the inhalants, oils and 'tickly cough' cures given under **Colds** and **Chest Infections** will work well.

Extra Answers

● *Essential oil of eucalyptus or pine* A few drops of either in hot water are good to inhale.

Spring Remedy
2 fresh young nettle tops
1 tablespoon blackberry leaves
1 sprig fresh peppermint
1 head meadowsweet
600ml(1 pint) boiling water

Infuse all the herbs in the boiling water for 10 minutes, covered. Take in the springtime to clear this painful problem before summer arrives.

CATARRHAL INFECTIONS

Catarrhal infections seem to be more rife today than ever before. In the past when one had a snorting cold one convalesced until it ran its course. Nowadays we rely on 'miracle cures' to dry up or stop these maladies instantly. We continue to work or send our children to school with blocked-up noses, headaches and coughs, armed with a bottle of magic, and wonder why after a week or so the infection returns, twice as potent and with the added pain of searing sinuses, ear-ache, tummy trouble, sickness, lethargy and downright tearful misery.

Catarrh can be the result of infection but it may also be a result of external irritations triggering an overproduction of mucus: dust, smoke, or an allergic reaction to certain foodstuffs, particularly milk and dairy produce, refined carbohydrates, fried food, nuts, grains and pulses and in some cases eggs, red meat and even oranges. If you or your family suffer consistently from catarrh try leaving out certain foodstuffs for several weeks at a time to check if they are the cause. A sluggish liver and constipation do not improve matters and nor does overeating, particularly of junk food. Stress may also be a factor. As well as the misery of painful sinuses which may make you feel very woozy and temporarily deplete your vision and cause ear-ache, loss of the senses of smell and taste, sore throat, coughs, sneezes and a runny nose, other unpleasant side effects which may result from persistent catarrh are bad breath and body odour, chronic constipation and spots.

Most of the remedies suggested for **Coughs** will help alleviate the misery of catarrhal infection and the dietary suggestions given for **Arthritis**, **Rheumatism** and **Constipation** will bring about a long-term improvement in the general state of health.

Inhalants and warm, pain-relieving oils rubbed on to the chest, throat and the areas surrounding the eyes and nose will help unblock nasal and respiratory passages. These are also to be found under **Coughs** and **Colds** but check first that they are suitable for use on the face.

Plenty of liquids, fresh fruits, green vegetables and keeping warm but not hot in a well ventilated room will all help to clear the infection completely and prevent it from escalating into something worse.

Most of these old-fashioned remedies suggested that steps to prevent and cure catarrhal infection could be more effective if started in warm weather. It would certainly do no harm to embark on a course of preventative action during the spring and summer months.

Gentle Remedies

● *Red rose petal and rose hip tea* Buy the ready-prepared tea as it has been rid of all the tiny irritant hairs. A regular glass night and morning relieves catarrh and bronchitis.

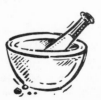

• *Marjoram, marsh mallow, melissa, vervain, borage or hyssop* These all make mildly antiseptic and delicious teas or infusions which will bring relief, promote gentle perspiration and soothe the throat. Add honey and a dash of lemon for enhanced benefit.

• *Yarrow tea* A tea which not only makes you feel a lot better but can also be used to wash and wipe itchy eyelids. This is very important when children's eyes are 'gummed up'. Use a separate piece of cotton wool for each eye and burn immediately after using.

• *Fenugreek tea* Drink it warm every morning throughout the year – 1 level teaspoon to 1 breakfast cup of water – to prevent catarrh from occurring. Sniff it up the nose when foresight did not prevail and you are stricken.

• *Aspirin* This is the old-fashioned remedy for catarrh and the only one which many practitioners believe actually works. Years ago the only satisfactory 'medicine' which would have been prescribed for this type of cold was the powdered bark of white willow or a tea of meadowsweet. Both of these herbs contain a high proportion of salicylic compound which is the basic constituent of aspirin.

Brutal Release

Perhaps the least delicious of the ancient remedies is to take duckweed boiled in a pan and throw upon it as much blood and butter as it will take. Eat hot to relieve the body of foul poisons. Not pleasant but reputedly a cure for catarrh, constipation and cramps.

• *Lemon juice* As well as featuring in the soothing drinks and gargles which we have come to expect – warm lemon juice well laced with cinnamon is a particularly helpful gargle and honey and lemon the best night-time drink – lemon juice may be sniffed neat and brutally up the nose, although you may prefer to dilute it in the proportions of the juice of ½ lemon to 300ml(½ pint) warm water. Inhale the strong vapours of the peel and juice of lemons steeped in boiling water whilst crouched beneath an all enveloping towel to relieve catarrhal congestion and prevent it from developing into sinusitis or ear-ache.

• *Boracic powder* Sniffed neat up the nose this is a very old-fashioned remedy. Alternatively mix together 15g(½oz) each of fine sea salt, baking soda and boracic powder in 600ml(1 pint) of warm water. Use this 1 tablespoon at a time diluted in 3 tablespoons of warm water to sniff up the nose at bedtime.

A Refreshing and Healthy Salad
1 crisp eating apple
3 dandelion leaves
1 fresh or dried fig
1 basil leaf
1 teaspoon fresh lemon juice
2 teaspoons olive oil
sea salt and freshly ground black
pepper to taste

Wash the apple well and chop it up without peeling. Make sure that the dandelions are clean and have been picked from an area free from contamination. Shred them and add them to the apple. Chop the fig. Mix together then add the lemon juice followed by the olive oil. Season well and eat immediately.

EAR-ACHE

Who amongst us has not at some time suffered from the sheer misery of ear-ache and felt aching sympathy when our own child has ear-ache? I have to admit that it is one of the very few childhood ailments which, if I cannot clear it myself within a few hours with the application of warm oil and aspirin and it has become progressively more painful, I have absolutely no compunction in calling for professional advice, even in the middle of the night.

Ear-ache can be caused by many things: colds, catarrh, 'flu, enlarged adenoids, infection caused by swimming in polluted water (which may also be the cause of an abscess in the ear), teething and wisdom teeth. Apart from the nasty, nagging agony of ear-ache there may also be dizziness and deafness which can indicate too much wax in the ears. If after using a gentle home remedy the ear-ache is not getting any better, if the bone underneath the ear is painful and the skin behind it is red and tender (but do make sure that this is not caused by ill-fitting spectacles), or if the patient has a stiff neck and is feeling drowsy it would be wise to seek immediate professional advice. Ear-ache does usually disappear quite quickly once it is treated but if it persists or keeps recurring over a period of time it is best to see your doctor.

Whilst there are some delightful remedies for ear-ache it is always wise to remember never to poke things into the ears, particularly garlic, onion or cotton wool buds on sticks. If an accident does occur and you realize that some foreign object has disappeared without trace into a small ear the Out Patient Department of your local hospital is the best place to deal with it. Do not try to remove it yourself. The local hospital are also very good at removing moths and spiders which creep into the ear at night and create enough mayhem within your head to convince you that the cavalry has taken up residence. You can actually try to drown and float these intruders out with warm oil but this is difficult to achieve if you live alone.

Most remedies for ear-ache are primarily based on warmth and oil but what lends such fascination to the subject is the quality and varieties of oils used throughout the world which have been tested and found satisfactory. Most importantly, the one thing that the majority of them have in common is the fact that none of the greases or oils used hardens on cooling. In England one would have caught a hedgehog, shaved off his prickles and roasted him slowly over a fire, catching the fat in a small pan as it dripped. In Europe the dormouse was the innocent victim whilst in Egypt the fine layer of fat from the portly hippopotamus was greatly sought after. Castor oil, butter, goose grease and chicken fat were also used more in the manner of emergency measures, although roasting limpets to extract the liquid would have needed a certain amount of foresight. Although many old-fashioned suggestions feature the use of roasted onion or garlic it is never wise to put solid substances in the ear but crushing either bulb and steeping it for several hours in warm oil before straining well through a fine gauze will give a healing unguent which has been used for centuries without ill effect. Many old encyclopaedias recommended warm honey or warm honey and garlic oil for a boil in the ear but I would think that this could lead to sticky complications. Garlic oil was also used by old-fashioned medics to relieve noises in the ears.

Ear-ache is often caused by water getting trapped in the ear during swimming and diving and, whilst I do not advocate 'head banging', a good shake of the head or holding the ear downwards and applying a firm but gentle massage underneath should release it.

To Soothe and Warm

Warmth is one of the greatest possible soothers and the methods of applying it have varied from heating a quantity of salt and rolling it in a cloth which is then placed in a sock upon which the aching ear is laid to hot poultices of onions, figs or hollyhocks (depending upon the region in which you lived) to draw out the pain. Camomile heads warmed by the fire, a fomentation of hot mustard leaf, hot pancakes and baked potatoes wrapped in wool have all been urged upon the unhappy sufferer, but the most sensible suggestions are those of a compress as hot as can be stood or a hot-water bottle well wrapped in a cover upon which to lay the painful ear whilst trying to sleep. Many people advocate another hot-water bottle at the feet no matter how warm the weather, presumably in an attempt to draw the pain as far from the ear as can be contrived! The most comforting warmth for any small child is mother's bosom and the type of crooning cuddle which will hopefully distract attention from the sore ear. Ear-ache in young children is often associated with teething troubles.

Massage can bring a great deal of relief especially if the cause of the pain is not certain. Massaging the gums behind the back teeth with oil of clove and cinnamon (not the essential oils) will ease pain related to the back teeth

coming through, particularly wisdom teeth. Dilute a few drops in almond oil for young children who may otherwise balk at the fieriness.

A gentle circular massage with the fingertips of the area of the face where it joins the ear will also ease ear-ache considerably, especially if one of the soothing, healing oils mentioned under **Chest Infections** is used. I have also found the magical Tiger balm to be an excellent emergency treatment.

- *Pleasant soothing herbal teas* All herbal teas, but especially summer savory, will help to relax and soothe the victim of ear-ache whilst basil tea will also relieve congestion and calm the spirit. The leaves of basil chewed fresh have double the potency.
- *Sweet almond oil* This is the most commonly used oil to ease ear-ache. Warm a teaspoon by plunging it into hot water. Shake it dry and quarter fill it with oil. Make the patient lie or sit with the painful ear upwards and tilted slightly back then check that the oil is not too hot and pour it gently into the ear, ensuring that it goes right in and does not trickle down the face. Massage very gently under the ear where it joins the cheek. Plug it with a large piece of cotton wool (countryfolk used sheep's wool because it was greasy and thick) to prevent the oil seeping out and to keep it warm. Olive oil can be used instead.
- *Parsley* Parsley oil or the juice from parsley applied on a substantial cotton wool plug is another old-fashioned remedy.
- *Essential oil of peppermint, cloves or calendula (marigold)* Add 1 drop of any one of these to 1 tablespoon of almond oil and use as above. Clove oil can also be used to clean the ears.
- *St John's wort oil (red oil)* This oil was one of the most important items on

a wise woman's inventory. Use as almond oil (above).

• *Lemon juice or onion juice* Applied to the offending ear on a plug of cotton wool, either of these should stop any infection immediately.

• *Ground ivy* An oil made from this delightful herb soothes ear-ache, cleans minor wounds and also makes an excellent rub on throat and neck when chesty colds are rampant. Take several good handfuls of the fresh, crushed plant and leave to stand in a jar filled with 600ml(1 pint) of olive or sunflower oil. Macerate for one month on a sunny windowsill, shaking occasionally, then strain through fine muslin before using.

• *Vitamin E oil or garlic oil capsules* The capsules are an excellent method of transporting a healing oil abroad for use when ear-ache occurs on holiday – which, because a lot of time is spent in the sea or swimming pools where water may be polluted, happens quite frequently. The great advantage is that the capsule can be pierced with a sterilized pin and the oil emptied directly into the ear if the teaspoon and hot water with which to warm it are not readily to hand.

SORE THROAT

A sore throat is usually attendant upon a cold and cough either as a result of tonsils being swollen or an infection and irritation in the throat which can also lead to ear-ache. It can, however, be caused by other illnesses, by tiredness or by too much speaking or shouting. It can also be the result of sleeping on your back with your mouth wide open or of smoking. Most old-fashioned remedies rely heavily upon gargling, sucking throat pastilles (this increases the flow of saliva and makes the throat

more comfortable) and keeping the neck and throat warm. Most of the remedies given for **Chest Infections** and **Colds** will improve this uncomfortable condition. You may prefer not to try the recommended cures of either wrapping a dirty sock around your neck, making sure that the heel is covering the larynx, or employing the services of a 'leech doctor'.

Gargles and Drinks

The correct way to gargle is to take a mouthful of the chosen solution, tilt the head back and, making sure that the liquid is right at the back of the throat, roll it in an 'ahh-hh-hh' sound. Tilting your head back and making a noise will close the throat and stop you swallowing. Gargle well for a good few seconds then spit out.

• *Sage gargle* Make a tea with 25g(1oz) fresh sage to 600ml(1 pint) of water and add $\frac{1}{4}$ teaspoon of cayenne. Leave to stand until cool. Strain through a fine sieve before using.

• *Red sage tea* Infuse 1 teaspoon of dried red sage in 1 cup of boiling water. Cover and leave for 10 minutes then strain and add a dash of vinegar. The tea, without the vinegar, can also be drunk $\frac{1}{2}$ cup at a time four times a day.

• *Thyme tea* Use both to gargle with and to drink.

• *Blackcurrant or blackberry jam* Either of these in a cup of hot water and strained before using is a good emergency gargle. So are blackcurrant juice and blackcurrant jelly, shrub, rob, cordial or vinegar, diluted in a cup of boiling water, with or without cinnamon added. They can all be used to gargle with and then drunk.

• *Lemon juice* Lemon and honey taken hot at night will do much to cure a sore throat and is one of the best remedies. Many people spray the back of the throat with neat lemon juice in an atomizer – you could try the same thing for children but use pure, fresh orange juice instead. One old-fashioned remedy suggests compresses of lemon to the throat. Take plenty of lemon or orange drinks made fresh as you need them, particularly lemon barley.

● *Cayenne and vinegar* Mix together 1 teaspoon of cayenne, 2 teaspoons of sea salt, 2 teaspoons of vinegar and 300ml($\frac{1}{2}$ pint) of warm water and use to gargle. Vinegar and warm water or salt diluted in warm water are old-fashioned gargles which always work well.

● *Glycerine and thymol* Use 1 part of this compound to 3 parts of warm water as a gargle.

● *Hydrogen peroxide* Add 1 dessert-spoon to $\frac{1}{2}$ tumbler of warm water and gargle.

● *Whisky and warm water* To be gargled with then drunk. Many people prefer to forego the water.

● *Syrup of figs* Dilute 1 teaspoon in $\frac{1}{2}$ cup of hot water and drink after gargling. There are a great many complex remedies, particularly from abroad, which use figs a great deal for curing a sore throat.

● *Pomegranate* The juice of fresh pomegranates is good to gargle with then to drink.

● *Creosote and aspirin* This is old-fashioned strong-man stuff *not* to be taken seriously.

Safeguards and Sweeteners

● *Neck scarves* All parents know that if you have a sore throat you must keep your neck warm.

● *Garlic oil, Olbas Oil or the essential oils of lemon, geranium, hyssop, sage or thyme* Diluted in almond, sunflower or olive oil these should be rubbed into the throat then covered with a warm scarf. They can also be dropped on to boiling water and the vapours inhaled through the open mouth.

● *Toast soaked in hot vinegar* The softened soggy toast should be sucked then swallowed.

● *Walnut husks stewed in honey* The strained syrup cures sore throats and tickly coughs.

● *Sunflower oil* One teaspoon taken neat cures sore throats and also works for loss of voice.

● *Sweet suckets* Most good quality natural or herbal throat pastilles will bring relief. So will barley sugar and butterscotch but best of all are your own home-made fruit pastilles (see page 134).

● *Tomatoes* Tinned tomatoes with vinegar sprinkled on them are one of the foods that children with painful throats can get down. Simmer them in a little olive oil and garlic and put them through a sieve if the pips are going to be troublesome.

● *Ice cream and jelly* These are always given to children who have had their tonsils out. Whilst ice cream is neither cheap nor easy to make at home I recommend that you try making your own jelly with pure fruit juices, honey and gelatine.

● *Angelica* Chew the candied stems of angelica to counteract a sore throat, but not just before bed-time as angelica is a mild stimulant and may keep you awake.

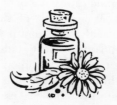

TONSILLITIS, LARYNGITIS AND PHARYNGITIS

These ailments are not really the same at all but are so closely connected that folk medicine makes small distinction. They are inflammation of the tonsils, the larynx and the pharynx respectively and are painful enough to make swallowing and breathing difficult. Laryngitis may result in loss of voice. The only real cure is to stay in bed and take aspirin every four hours. If the condition does not clear up within two days or if it recurs frequently seek professional advice. Most of the remedies given within the sections on **Chest Infections** and **Colds, Sneezing and Influenza** will bring some relief.

To Relieve and Cure

● *Vinegar* Wrapping the throat with a rag soaked in warm vinegar appears to be the most popular suggestion to ease the pain of all sore throats.
● *Garlic, onion or leek* Drunk either in a broth or chewed raw, any of these would certainly help to clear the system of infection.
● *Slippery elm* Mix 3 teaspoons of the powdered bark to a paste with 1 teaspoon of cayenne, 2 teaspoons of

clear honey and 4 teaspoons of warm water. Take by the teaspoon as needed.
● *Fig and honey syrup* Drink the syrup from dried figs steeped in just enough water to cover then stewed with honey. This is recommended for laryngitis and hoarseness.
● *Mallow flowers, althea root, liquorice root, mullein, coltsfoot and pimpernel* Mix together 1 tablespoon of each of these and take 1 teaspoon at a time in ½ cup of boiling water sweetened with honey.
● *Elderflowers* Inhale the vapours of dried elderflowers in boiling water to ease laryngitis and reduce hoarseness.
● *Lavender* Infuse 25g(1oz) in 1 litre(1¾ pints) of boiling water for five minutes. Gargle with this infusion. Lavender or elderflower vinegar diluted with hot water are other good gargles.
● *Rose petal jelly* Taken by the teaspoon this is an effective remedy for tonsillitis (see page 93).

A Recipe To Improve Hoarseness and Loss of Voice
450g(1lb) strong onions
50g(2oz) honey
350g(12oz) brown sugar
1 litre(1¾ pints) water

Peel and chop the onions very finely. Combine the ingredients and cook gently for three hours. Pot into dry sterilized jars. Seal and keep refrigerated. Take 4 tablespoons a day.

GLANDULAR PROBLEMS

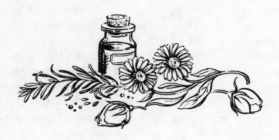

When I attended my first kindergarten we were introduced to the workings of the body so that we might assimilate some knowledge of hygiene and first aid. On the board a life-sized figure depicted the glands as soldiers fighting a vanguard action against the invasion of illness which, although oversimplified, is correct for although adding to our discomfort when we are ill they do have this purpose.

Glands in the throat may swell up when there is an ear, nose and throat infection or as a result of bad teeth, whilst swollen glands under the arm or in the groin may be caused by an infected cut, bite or sting on arms or legs – in which case it should be examined professionally. Persistently swollen glands in any part of the body should not be ignored.

Any disruptions in the normal functioning of the thyroid, prostate and lymph glands require professional attention.

GLANDULAR FEVER

This is a viral disease which antibiotics will not 'cure' and although it is fairly common it can be unpleasant and recurring. The symptoms are similar to influenza but with swollen glands and occasionally a rash. If you have what you think is 'flu but with the above symptoms for longer than a week seek professional advice. You must stay indoors and rest and not go back to school or work until completely fit. As with all feverish illnesses depression and a general feeling of listlessness may follow glandular fever. It is important that you take plenty of liquids, particularly water or orange, lemon or grape juice.

142

Old-Fashioned Suggestions for Bringing Comfort

Tincture of iodine was at one time painted on to the swollen glands or they were covered with warm red flannel. There used to be a great concern that the afflicted area should not be allowed to 'catch cold'.

● *Grapes* Grape poultice is used in some parts of the world to ease the pain of swollen glands but I think that the following soothing drink is probably of more benefit.

Grape Barley Water
3¾ litres(6 pints) home-made barley water (see page 126)
225g(8oz) honey
350ml(12 fl oz) bottled grape juice

Strain the barley water when it is cool and mix with the other ingredients. Bottle and store in the refrigerator. Shake before using. If you like you can double the amounts of honey and grape juice used.

● *Mullein* Use as a compress on swollen glands or drink as a tea.

● *Bayberry* Gargle with an infusion of the leaves.
● *Walnut* Macerate 50g(2oz) of walnut leaves in 1 litre(1¾ pints) of cold water for two hours. Bring gently to the boil and boil for two minutes then infuse for 15 minutes. Use on cloths to poultice swollen glands. The pounded leaf was also laid on the painful area to bring relief.
● *Dandelion, nettle or horse's tail tea* All of these teas made in the proportions of 25g(1oz) to 600ml(1 pint) of water are reputed to bring relief to those suffering from a disturbance of the thyroid gland. Take by the small cup every three hours, sweetened with honey.
● *Sea food, kelp tablets, runner beans, agar-agar and garlic* All of these are recommended additions to the diet for those suffering from goitre (enlargement of the thyroid).
● *Bladderwrack tea* A tea made from 25g(1oz) of bladderwrack to 600ml(1 pint) of water can be applied externally or drunk (½ cup diluted with water) before retiring to bed for thyroid problems.
● *Parsley, watercress and molasses* Anyone suffering from thyroid disturbances will find these invaluable additions to their diet.

IRRITATIONS OF THE EYES

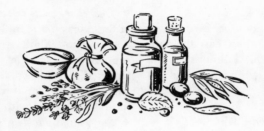

There are many minor ways in which the eyes can become afflicted and which may not require professional advice and the most common of these are soreness, tiredness and irritation, conditions which are easily identified and dealt with.

Pollen, dust and dirt are the tiny infiltrators which can make one's eyes smart and tickle, whilst larger foreign bodies such as lashes, pieces of leaf and insects can create quite different problems which will require the help of a friend to turn back the eyelid and remove the culprit with the corner of a clean white cloth. Do not poke around in the eye looking for the irritant. Either the naturally produced tears or an eye-bath will wash it away without any further damage being done although the eye will continue to feel as though there is a chunk of brick embedded in it. A good blow of the nose will often relieve irritation and weeping eyes. If you are unable to remove a foreign substance, particularly something dangerously

nasty – a metal shaving or a thorn – you should go immediately to the Out Patient Department of your nearest hospital. They can usually deal with it speedily and effectively thus preventing further damage and infection.

The best lotion for eyes mildly irritated by external causes is a gentle solution of warm boiled water and boracic crystals. Two drops of tincture of euphrasia (eyebright) or calendula (marigold) to 1 eyebath of warm boiled water are both very effective. A very old-fashioned idea which brought tremendous relief to itchy eyes, particularly to sufferers from hayfever, and which is now impractical because of pollution was to use sea water. The following eye lotion, however, is a happy alternative. Leave 600ml(1 pint) of water to stand uncovered overnight. The next day boil it and add 2 level teaspoons of sea salt, stirring well to dissolve. Cool and pour into a sterilized bottle and use to bathe the eyes. Whenever you use an eyebath make sure that it is very clean: this means plunging it in boiling water and shaking it dry. Use it on one eye only and repeat the cleaning process before using it again on the other eye.

SORE EYES

Sore eyes which continually give pain and irritation, are sensitive to sunlight, occasionally blur or water frequently may be the result of an allergy – examine the cause for this, particularly in respect to eye make-up. A lack of vitamin B$_2$ may also be the reason for these problems occurring. Two methods of relieving sore eyes are to bathe the lids with cold water and to cover the lids with cold compresses several times a day and at night. Do not rub the eyes when they are painful but instead close them and roll the eyes up, down and around under the lids.

TIRED EYES

This ambiguous description may cover many aspects from headache to blurred or poor vision. There is no doubt that a poor diet, stress, smoking, lack of sleep, straining the eyes by reading, writing, drawing or doing any close work in a poor light over a prolonged period of time and using modern V.D.U. equipment in the wrong conditions will all reduce our clarity of vision. If you are at all worried take professional advice but remember that stronger and stronger spectacles may not necessarily be the only option available – many authorities believe that the eyesight can be

improved by diet, exercise and a reorganized lifestyle.

Many of the eyewashes and compresses on pages 146–7 will soothe and reduce under eye puffiness, dark circles and bags.

EYE INFECTIONS

Conjunctivitis is an inflammation of the mucous membrane of the eye which can be caused by an allergy, hayfever, a foreign body in the eye or an infection. The eye becomes red and feels gritty and tired. It will water and the lids will irritate and become swollen and flaky. There is occasionally also an unpleasant discharge. To reduce the chance of this occurring take scrupulous care to wash the hands before and after touching the eyes.

Always keep cosmetic brushes, pencils and sponges immaculately clean and do not use eye make-up if you have an eye infection. If you use an eyebath sterilize it after each eye has been bathed. Use separate compresses of cotton wool for cleaning and soothing one eye at a time and discard immediately after using – preferably burn them. If suffering from conjunctivitis it is sensible to seek professional advice, especially in the case of children.

Styes are similar to a slowly developing boil on the upper lid or lower rim of the eye and are often a sign of general debility or, in old-fashioned parlance, 'being run down'. They are incredibly painful and can make you feel very low indeed. For a long-term improvement in health look to the diet and eat plenty of fresh green salads, fruit and strong green vegetables such as spinach.

An infusion of eyebright in milk was used to bathe sore eyes but it is better applied in a lotion of 2 drops of tincture of eyebright (euphrasia) to 2 tablespoons of rose water and 1 tablespoon of plain warm boiled water. Although this makes a soothing eyebath it is more effective when soaked into a cotton wool compress. A poultice of fresh steamed cabbage leaves or grated raw potato were two old-fashioned remedies calculated to bring about the speedy dispersal of a stye and so was a bread and milk poultice – in other words, any warm fomentation which would have a 'drawing' effect upon the stye and bring it to a head.

I can remember vividly from my own childhood that the three main remedies which were used to cure a stye in our household were an eyebath of warm boracic lotion, a bearably hot cotton wool compress (over which we needlessly complained) and a perfectly magical unguent called Golden Eye Ointment which was, I believe, also known as Pulsatilla. However when my mother was not looking my grandmother would slip in to rub the afflicted lid with her golden wedding ring which she swore was the only foolproof remedy. Thank heavens that she had not heard of the one involving the powdered bones of a haddock!

Honourable Eyewashes and Compresses

● *Tea bags* Ordinary Indian tea, camomile tea or red raspberry leaf tea bags are all very soothing if laid warm upon the closed lids. They will help relieve the pain of a stye and reduce undereye puffiness. If the tea bags are not easily obtainable saturate cotton wool pads in the tea. Rose hip tea bags and papaya tea bags are those most popularly recommended by beauticians to get rid of 'bags under the eyes'. Another old favourite of the beauty parlour was to lay half a freshly cut fig

on the offending sags and bags to magically remove them.
● *Witch hazel* Make cooling compresses with refrigerated witch hazel to lay on the eyelids but make sure that it is used only externally as it can smart very painfully if it infiltrates beneath the lid. Used under the eyes it will reduce puffiness.
● *Honey* Take 600ml(1 pint) of boiling water, 1 handful of eyebright and 3 tablespoons of honey. Pour the water over the eyebright and leave until cool. Strain then dissolve the honey in the infusion. Soak cotton wool pads in this solution and leave them on the eyes for 20 minutes to relieve soreness. This remedy was also believed to improve the eyesight.
● *Elderflower water, eyebright or fennel infusions* Use one of these to bathe the lids when eyes are sore. They are particularly useful remedies if you have managed to burn your eyelids in the sun.
● *Lavender* One drop each of essential oils of lavender and lemon to 1 teaspoon of boiled water used to bathe the eye externally will ease conjunctivitis, styes and inflamed eyelids.
● *Chickweed, tansy or watercress* A handful of any one of these green goodies, simmered in a covered pan with 1 cupful of water or milk for five minutes then cooled, will make a healing lotion for external use on the eyelids. Strained of excess liquid and placed between muslin, all three herbs will also provide soothing warm or cold compresses for eyes tired from overwork, central heating or air conditioning – all of which create a feeling of dryness and tension.
● *Potatoes* Grated raw potato has been used a great deal to ease sore puffy eyelids and reduce undereye puffiness. Either strain the juice from a grated

potato and saturate cotton wool pads with it or lay the grated vegetable on the eye between layers of muslin. Slices of raw potato or a compress of 1 tablespoon of crushed nasturtium seed added to 1 tablespoon of grated potato will soothe swollen eyelids and reduce swelling – this is a handy tip if you like to indulge in a good cry. A few tears are good for the eyes but we are told that too many will weaken them.

• *Apples* A sparkle can be brought back to lacklustre eyes by the following method. Infuse 1 tablespoon of marigold petals in 125ml(4 fl oz) of boiling water. Strain the liquid then simmer 1 peeled and finely chopped apple in it. When it is soft, drain the apple, allow to cool and when of a comfortable temperature lay it between two layers of gauze. Place on the eyes and leave for 10 minutes. Apple juice which is smooth, silky and rich in pectin can also be used to wipe sore eyes but it must be juice which has been extracted from cooked apple otherwise it will smart too much. A poultice of raw, grated apple has been considered the only method of reducing bruising caused by a blow in the eye.

• *Carrots* A lack of vitamin A can cause poor night vision and as carrots contain a goodly amount of carotene, which is converted to this vitamin in the liver, a large quantity of them in the diet was considered to be the definitive answer. A diet which also includes apricots, peaches, good dark green leafy vegetables, red peppers, cod liver oil, prunes, beetroot, egg yolk and butter is even healthier and more sensible. Many old-fashioned diets recommended that peaches and apricots were absolute necessities to improve failing vision associated with debility, and I feel sure such a diet would have been the prerogative of the fairly well to do and only

obtainable in sun-soaked countries and it would seem likely that a winter spent in the sunshine would certainly perk up all one's faculties. Most 'golden' things were considered to be beneficial to the sight but one of the nicest thoughts is that to gaze upon the bright marigold each day would improve vision. It would undoubtedly make you feel more cheerful.

• *Mint* The juice from freshly crushed mint leaves will help eradicate dark shadows beneath the eyes.

• *Castor oil* A minute amount of perfectly fresh castor oil smeared along the lids will reduce flaky swelling and irritation but like all oils you should not get it into the eye for it will smart. One tablespoon of castor oil mixed with 2 tablespoons of almond oil is an excellent eye make-up remover.

• *Almond, apricot and coconut oils* All of these are good for lubricating the delicate skin around the eyes. Frequent, gentle massage will help to arrest and disperse fine lines (see below).

The Gentle Touch

Do not rub sore, tired and irritating eyes for not only might you damage them but they will become red and swollen and you will drag the surrounding soft skin. Try instead the following methods of relieving discomfort.

• *Palming* Press the base of the palms of the hands gently but firmly over the closed lids and maintain pressure for several minutes.

• *Blinking* Blink the eyes several times in rapid succession. Close the eyes and go through the same blinking movements.

• *Sunning* A little but not too much sun on the eyelids helps to strengthen the eyes but never look into the sun.

● *Massage* Using a little fine oil and the tips of three fingers stroke gently from the bridge of the nose out across the eyes beneath and above the brow several times. With finger and thumb pinch the nose beneath the bridge and maintain the pressure for several seconds then using one finger make a stroking movement from the bridge of the nose, across the cheek, under the eyes to the temple.

These massage movements bring tremendous relief when sinus problems are causing the eyes to ache and when a headache is present. In this instance cold compresses on the region of the eyes and nose will also help to bring relief.

Nervous Disorders

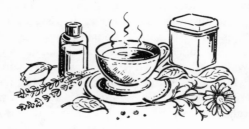

Two of my favourite books are an old-fashioned American 'Homesteading Manual' and an early 20th century encyclopaedia designed to help young housewives. Neither of these books however is very forthcoming on the subject of nervous disorders and nor, I notice, are the otherwise forthright herbals of yesteryear, although many of the remedies given for identifiable illnesses were no more or less than tranquillizers and sedatives. There appeared to be little time then for 'imaginary ailments' amongst hard-working families, but fashionable little brews and tisanes were to be found in abundance in those treatises offered up by wily gentlemen who dallied with the frayed nerves of society ladies.

One does not suffer from illnesses which have their roots in imaginary causes when one is too busy to dwell on them. However the stresses which the latter half of this century inflicts upon us, although less physically demanding, are nonetheless just as damaging as those suffered by our forefathers. Before the days of psychological assessments an illness was treated for what it was without looking for underlying causes but it has to be said that many genuine physical problems such as palpitations, stomach ache, depression, insomnia and nightmares, skin eruptions, breathing difficulties, sweating, tearfulness, phobia and needless panic, even all the aches and pains associated with backache and arthritis may be as much due to mental as to physical stress.

ANXIETY

We should be able to take most worries in our stride without becoming unduly anxious but if we get to the point where we feel physically wretched, where problems loom terrifyingly in our minds by day and pursue us relentlessly into our dreams by night, it is time to take stock of the situation. Irrational anxiety may have a purely physical cause such as a poor diet leading to a deficiency of minerals and vitamins. Low blood sugar level or too many stimulants in the form of coffee, tea and cigarettes can also contribute to a feeling of impending doom. Inevitably the worse we feel the worse we become. Holding ourselves taut and strung out with tension can create difficulties in breathing; it makes muscles ache, the jaw stiff, the neck rigid and we may suffer from stomach pains. We slump into a depressed posture which causes indigestion and constipation. Nervous tensions, stress and strain not only upset the digestive system but may also interfere with the hormonal balance of the body. We become tired, our faces become drawn and indented with anxious lines and we look and therefore feel doubly dreadful.

All the unpalatable platitudes which were meant to stop us feeling sorry for ourselves can be crystallized into several very commonsensical suggestions.

Take some regular exercise in which the mind has to become totally absorbed in what you are doing and thoughts cannot wander – a quick and unaccustomed jog around the block whilst your mind is busy beavering unhappily away will not do.

When an anxious, aggressive, fearful or negative thought burrows randomly into your consciousness briskly disperse it with a pleasant picture of your own choosing and work hard elaborating on that. Refuse to allow yourself to dwell upon beastly thoughts, especially those inflicted upon you, willy nilly, by the media. The days are gone when we might have collected the leaves of heliotrope in which we could wrap bay leaves and a wolf's tooth to protect ourselves against cruel thoughts and unkind words.

Relaxation or learning to relax, taking long controlled breaths, practising yoga or meditation, swimming or walking with a purpose (birdwatching, admiring other folks' gardens) will all help to dispel anxiety. So will a long chat into a friendly ear. One of the best methods of relaxing is to have a massage or to visit a reflexologist and have your feet massaged – this is something that you can do for yourself at home and it will make you feel immeasurably better, as will having your back, shoulders and neck massaged, especially if, with practise, you can manage to induce in yourself a trance-like state. I have heard it said that in order to achieve this one must turn one's third eye inwards.

Essential oils are some of the best remedies for reducing tension. Use them in a carrier oil to massage the body or throw a few drops into a warm bath. The following are those most frequently recommended to relieve tension and stress: basil, marjoram, fennel, hyssop, rosemary, thyme, tarragon and sage. If the hormonal balance is affected both drinking sage tea and massaging with essential oil of sage are particularly effective. All of these herbs should be taken in tea and used lavishly in cooking too. Bergamot, camomile, juniper, lavender, vervain and orange can also be used as essential oils in bath and massage and the herbs used in tea as a mild sedative and digestive. Coriander, geranium, neroli, cedarwood and frankincense are spicy healing oils which are particularly calming when used in the bath.

There are very few old-fashioned remedies to relieve anxiety beyond suggesting that one eats plenty of brown bread, wheatgerm, molasses, honey, milk and oats. Self-help is by far the best remedy for anxiety. Although not initially an easy answer, once you have learned the lesson it is always there for you to fall back on in a crisis and although habit-forming it is not detrimental to the health.

Soothing Drinks

In addition to those given below, any of the relaxing and soothing herb teas suggested elsewhere in this book will help.

- *Warm milk and honey with a dash of cinnamon* This is the best drink to take at night both to help you relax and to stave off insomnia.
- *Honey* Take by the spoonful or in hot water whenever tired and low.
- *Hop tea* Three hop cones or heads in 1 cup of boiling water taken the moment you begin to feel excessively tense is a marvellous remedy for anxiety and insomnia.

A Tea to Soothe and Heal
the Troubled Spirit
25g(1oz) each dried camomile flowers, linden blossom (lime flowers), hibiscus blossoms and marigold flowers
15g(½oz) each dried peppermint leaves and vervain
1 teaspoon whole fenugreek seeds
100g(4oz) Lapsang Souchong
tea

Mix all the ingredients together and store in a dark airtight container. Use 1 teaspoon to 300ml(½ pint) of boiling water in a tea pot and leave to stand for five minutes before straining and serving with a slice of lemon and 1 teaspoon of honey if liked. This tea calms turmoil and anxiety and also helps to clear a fuzzy head and upset tummy. One cup morning and night will sustain a feeling of well-being.

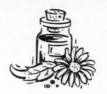

A Tea to Soothe the Nerves
1 teaspoon each grated dried valerian root and dried mint
½ teaspoon each dried camomile and lavender flowers
600ml(1 pint) boiling water

Infuse the dry ingredients in the water for 15 minutes then strain and take 1 glass three times a day for one week only.

- *Two tonic teas to take when feeling low* Sip either 2 teaspoons of dandelion and 1 of basil infused in 600ml(1 pint) of boiling water or 2 teaspoons each of nettle, basil and melissa infused in 600ml(1 pint) of boiling water.

A Tonic Tea to Relieve Stress,
Anxiety and Debility
1 tablespoon each fresh dandelion and nettle tops
1 teaspoon each fresh blackcurrant and borage leaves
600ml(1 pint) of boiling water

Steep the greenery in the water for five minutes. Strain and drink with lemon and honey.

- *A good healthy breakfast* Oats are particularly strengthening and calm the nerves, making them a very good breakfast for youngsters who are taking exams. Take 1 tablespoon of raw oats, mix with 3 tablespoons of cold water and leave to stand for 12 hours. Blend with 1 tablespoon of lemon juice, 3 tablespoons of plain live yoghurt, 1 teaspoon of honey, 1 well-washed grated apple and a few chopped nuts. Oats can also of course be eaten as porridge. If you cannot get your offspring to eat breakfast get them to take a handful or bar of oaty health food with them to school. Muesli is another excellent breakfast and snack food.

The Nice Breakfast Food
450g(1lb) porridge oats
450g(1lb) fat juicy raisins
225g(8oz) wheatflakes
100g(4oz) wheatgerm
100g(4oz) mixed chopped nuts (not peanuts)
100g(4oz) crushed dried banana chips
100g(4oz) sesame seeds
50g(2oz) pumpkin seeds
50g(2oz) sunflower seeds

Mix all the ingredients together and serve with chopped fresh fruit, stewed dried fruit, yoghurt or milk. This makes enough to last a family several weeks.

● *Flapjack* There are many really good recipes using oats, honey, dates, walnuts and so on. Not only and in every possible way is flapjack preferable to jam doughnuts but it is also an easily carried form of pure goodness – nourishing, sustaining and one of the few snacks to be recommended for eating before bed. Flapjack helps insomniacs and reduces the chance of nightmares, especially in children.

DEBILITY

When we feel tired, listless, lacking in energy and downhearted it is quite frequently related to stress but more often it is a result of poor nutrition caused by too many convenience and junk foods, ill-advised dieting or loss of appetite which, again, may be the result of tension. Hormonal imbalance causing water retention which is distressing, depressing and thus debilitating and eating poorly regulated or inadequate meals can create this problem. Therefore in the first instance look to the diet whilst trying to build a gentle routine of exercise and make sure that you get enough rest. If you still feel consistently below par take professional advice, some of which will probably be that you need a holiday or a good tonic – ginseng is an old favourite.

Eat plenty of salads and dark green vegetables. Watercress was thought to be the most beneficial to combat debility and the young fresh roots of horse's tail (equisetum) eaten raw were considered not only to improve a nervous spirit and do you good but to taste better than asparagus. Other tonic herbs to shred into a salad are parsley, salad burnet, sorrel, sweet cicely, chives, chickweed, caraway and chervil. The green cocktail, sunset slinger and many of the salads mentioned in this book will also improve the general state of health.

● *Dock* This was used as one of the great tonic herbs as it has a very high iron content. You might like to try this old-fashioned dock wine as an alternative to commercial brands.

Dock Wine
175g(7oz) dock root
15g(½oz) liquorice wood
7g(¼oz) juniper berries
100g(4oz) raw cane sugar
2 litres(3½ pints) robust (non-chemical) red wine

Put all the ingredients together in a china container, cover and place either in a very slow oven or in a bain-marie.

Continue to heat gently until the mixture is reduced by half. Strain, bottle and seal tightly. Drink 1 sherry glass each morning for two weeks.

● *Rosemary in wine* Steep 6 sprigs of rosemary in 1 bottle of sweet white wine for 14 days and keep sealed. Take 1 wineglass as a daily tonic.

DEPRESSION

From anxiety springs depression which, some say, is like a great black beast that dogs your footsteps everywhere you go. To others it is the heavy black bird hunched immovably on your shoulder. Some people cure it with sleep and others by taking a bottle of whisky beneath the table. For those who have not suffered it there is no way to describe the mood of meaningless black despair.

Minor despair or glumness of the spirit can be mitigated however. Often it is as a result of a vitamin B (particularly B$_6$) deficiency or it may be an allergy which triggers an unhappy reaction. Some people suffer from acute depression after taking antibiotics. If you realize that what appeared to be only a bad case of 'down in the dumps' is becoming fearsome find someone to chat to. Do not take tranquillizers for they are not the answer.

Non-Addictive Answers

A brisk walk before breakfast and meditation are both well worth making time for, and so is a warm bath at night using any one of the essential oils suggested to soothe **Anxiety**.

● *Apple cider vinegar and honey* Take 1 tablespoon of vinegar in a small wineglass of warm water with a little honey, first thing in the morning and last thing at night.

● *Orange juice* Drink orange juice each morning, especially if it is made fresh using the whole fruit. There is something particularly soothing in taking the time to make your own at breakfast each day.

● *Rosemary and sage* Use plenty of these herbs in cooking and drink either in a herbal tea.

● *Chervil* Use it in salads for it is reputed to brighten the spirit.

● *Walnuts* It was believed that their convoluted shape resembled, therefore must be helpful to, a poorly and fatigued brain. So eat plenty of them.

● *Herbal teas* Infuse 1 teaspoon of any of the following in 1 cup of boiling water: camomile, lemon balm, catnip, vervain, valerian.

● *Lavender* Place a lavender pillow beneath the head at night.

● *Marigolds* Grow pots of this bright flower on windowsill and patio. It gladdens the eye and cheers the spirit.

FAINTING AND DIZZINESS

Unnerving though it may be, fainting and falling flat on one's face is nature's way of restoring the circulation of blood to the brain, starvation of the latter having caused the dizziness and ultimately the faint in the first place. It is obviously more sensible to sit down as soon as you feel the warning signs of wobbly legs, dizziness and cold clamminess, for falling heavily can cause injury especially to the elderly. If you cannot lie down with your legs raised slightly sit with your head dropped firmly between your knees. There are many reasons why we faint. Sometimes it is shock, emotion or upset. It may be pain or plain exhaustion which causes us to

153

keel over, especially after standing for long periods in the heat – think of all those guardsmen who have succumbed over the years. We have all at some time or another experienced that unpleasantly disorientated feeling creeping over us and have made rapidly for a safe seat.

The immediate help for anyone who either feels faint or has fainted is to make sure that ties and tight clothing are loosened and that they are either sitting or lying down as suggested above. Old-fashioned remedies which always work wonderfully well are to rub the temples and hands with eau de Cologne or lavender water and to hold it beneath the nose, or to tap quickly and firmly with one fingernail on the small area beneath the centre of the nose and above the top lip. We used to call it tickling and sometimes a feather was used but the result was always the same. Pinching and slapping the hands was another favourite and also fanning the victim with anything that came to hand. I can also remember the stench of burning feathers held under the nose and the eye-stinging shock of smelling salts which contained ammonia, lavender, bergamot, rosemary and peppermint. In reality once the blood has returned to the brain the patient usually recovers but should nevertheless be kept warm and quiet for a while and given a few sips of either cold water or hot, sweet tea. A few drops of sal volatile (aromatic spirits of ammonia) in a wineglass of water was at one time the answer for hysteria, fainting and dizziness.

Gentle Restoratives

- *Peppermint, sage, lemon balm or rosemary tea* A tea made in the proportions of 25g(1oz) to 600ml(1 pint) of boiling water and sweetened with unrefined sugar or honey will speed recovery. Spirit of balm was the ancient remedy for all problems connected with the consciousness.
- *Cinnamon and honey* One dessertspoon of honey to 1 pinch of cinnamon in 1 cup of hot water is an excellent restorative.
- *Angelica* Considered by wise men to be the elixir of long life, it was often recommended in tonic form as a restorative for those suffering from fainting fits, weakness of the spirit and for convalescents. However as it can overstimulate do not take it too often and never at night. Children who feel weak, dizzy and below par will feel better if they chew a small piece of candied angelica.
- *Rosemary in wine* This should be taken to remedy mental overstrain (see page 153).
- *Lemon juice and honey* Take this mixture when giddiness starts.
- *Beetroot juice* It is believed that this will cure brain fatigue and giddiness.

HYSTERIA

Hysteria usually follows after a shock, whether physical or mental, severe or otherwise. The most important thing to remember is to remain calm and to be kind yet firm, strongly resisting the temptation to scream yourself or to slap the victim's face, a measure which can be taken only as a truly last resort. Dr Bach's Rescue Remedy is a very useful thing to keep in the house and has been known to quiet and calm the most profoundly shocked person and also hysterical animals. See also the section of this book on **Shock**.

To prevent hysteria taking a hold and manifesting itself later in a mental or physical condition try to make the patient lie down, give them a soothing tisane and try to get them to talk until eventually the experience is relived and expelled. Suppression can lead to physical illness. Hopefully they will then sleep and awake restored. Youngsters who become hysterical during exams and as a result of emotional upheavals can be helped in much the same way.

Calming Tisanes

- *Lady's bedstraw* Steep 25g(1oz) in 1 litre(1¾ pints) of boiling water.
- *Marigold* Steep 25g(1oz) in 1 litre (1¾ pints) of boiling water.
- *Valerian* Leave 15g(½oz) to macerate in 1 cup of cold water for 12 hours. Take 1 tablespoon if and when the patient appears to be getting 'in a state' again.

INSOMNIA

Many influences contribute to insomnia or the inability to sleep. Nervous tension, anxiety and illness are factors that may keep us awake at night but it is more likely that the problem lies with an uncomfortable bed or a room that is too hot or too cold or an intrusive light shining into the bedroom. Indigestion can cause you to wake several hours after dropping off whilst tension, depression or kidney problems may waken you in the early hours of the morning, after which sleep may elude you. Not being able to fall asleep easily or waking during the night or too early

upsets the complex sleep patterns which the body is accustomed to and leaves you tired, irritable and unable to concentrate. Do not take sleeping tablets for they will complicate matters further. Herbal sleeping tablets however are non-addictive and may be used to help regulate sleep patterns in an emergency.

Improve your diet which may need an additional supplement of vitamin B or calcium and cut out obvious stimulants such as coffee, tea and cigarettes, particularly at night-time. Do not watch television programmes late at night which may overexcite either the imagination or the brain – it is far better to take a good book to bed with you or one that is so mindlessly boring that you fall asleep trying to concentrate. On the whole I find this better than counting sheep. Other people find that concentrating on something mundane, such as tomorrow's menu, item for item, spoon by spoon in order of use, skipping nothing until in their mind the meal is on the table will send them to sleep. Others recite the longest poem they can recall. Most sufferers of night-time waking agree that nothing is to be gained by tossing and turning and cursing their misfortune and that the best cure is calm acceptance, a warm drink and a good book.

Physical Suggestions to Promote Sleep

John Wesley advocated a cold bath before retiring which makes you wonder what thoughts he feared might keep him awake at night! A warm bath is far more pleasant if it is scented with one of the following essential oils: camomile, sandalwood, lavender, rosemary, melissa, meadowsweet, orange, neroli, rose. All of these will calm a rest-

155

less spirit. Another somniferous idea is to hold a bathbag containing 3 parts camomile, 2 parts each meadowsweet and lime flowers and 1 part grated valerian root beneath the hot tap whilst the water is running.

A warm footbath is a comforting way of persuading the blood to rush from the head which many people believe is the best condition for sleep, although others swear the opposite and that the foot of the bed should be raised. I believe that a soothing herbal footbath does help you to sleep and my favourite is a mixture of lavender, rosemary and crushed juniper berries tied into a cotton handkerchief. More stalwart characters might prefer a mustard footbath.

Babies and young children who have difficulty sleeping or who suffer from nightmares might be soothed with the addition to their warm bath water of a strong tea made with camomile, lime flowers or lemon balm.

After a bath or footbath gently massage the whole body or feet with 3 drops of one of the essential oils suggested above mixed into a small cup of a base oil (such as a light vegetable oil). Not only will this promote sleep but it will also improve the condition of the skin.

The natives of parts of Italy were reputed to sleep with cloves of garlic between their toes or to rub their feet with garlic oil to ensure a sound night's sleep but I suspect their sleeplessness might have had more to do with their dread of vampires than an unquiet mind. Anointing the body with copious amounts of basil oil assured a dreamless sleep and one free from nightmares but unless you make your own basil oil use instead a few drops of essential oil of basil in olive oil.

Washing the head in dill water and placing bunches of dill upon the pillow was another method for curing insomnia and eating dill or drinking dillwater relieves indigestion which may be the cause of sleeplessness in the first place.

Where to place the bed seems to figure prominently in old wives' tales – turning it so that the head faces true north seems to be the favoured position and it is one adopted by many sensible and otherwise logical people. Less so the theory that your shoes should be placed upside down with the toes facing the head of the bed. Sleeping on your back is advocated to avoid nightmares but the sound of your snoring will keep everyone else awake. Deep-breathing exercises before you get into bed are a popular regimen, the preferred method being to breathe in through the mouth and exhale through the nose – a discipline which forces relaxation.

Old-fashioned remedies which have been well brought up to date are eating passion flowers, ground bones or pollen. Many primitive peoples set great store by a good night's sleep being convinced that were it otherwise their souls would leave their bodies and be lost to the night, never to return. Today if we wake feeling like zombies we may look for help in the form of passiflora, calcium, honey or pollen. Many people of my grandmother's generation swore by extract of oats as a method of calming an overactive mind but believed in their hearts that if you had done your day's work well, sleep would come easily.

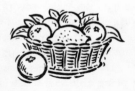

Bedtime Drinks

Do not drink copiously before retiring to bed, otherwise you will inevitably be awoken during the night.

- *Oranges* Orange flower water taken on a lump of sugar or in a little warm sweetened water is the most old-fashioned remedy for a multitude of anxiety-based problems. All gentlewomen kept a small flask on their bedside tables – a far better habit than some modern bedside bottles. Orange leaf tea or the juice of 2 oranges in a little hot water sweetened with honey are both pleasant night-time drinks which will remedy mild insomnia.
- *Milk or buttermilk* Drink either of these hot with a pinch of cinnamon and honey.
- *Hops* Infuse 3 tablespoons in 1 cup of boiling water. A hop pillow is a great sleep inducer and so is an old-fashioned and delightful 'dream pillow' filled with woodruff, lady's bedstraw and meadowsweet which has the sweet, clean smell of sun-dried hay. It is no wonder that folklore tells the tale that Mary gave birth to Jesus on a pallet of bedstraw – hence its name.
- *Lemon balm, melilot, mint or lime* These all make calming, soporific infusions.
- *A stronger herbal* Take 1 tablespoon each of dried or 1 handful of fresh red clover heads, shredded lettuce and hops. Place in 600ml(1 pint) of cold water, heat gently until boiling and boil for two minutes. Simmer for a further two then remove from the heat. Infuse for three hours. Strain and bottle. Well sealed it will keep in a cool dark place for up to four days. Take a small glassful at night to help you sleep.
- *Catnip, lemon balm or camomile* Small children and babies who have difficulty in getting to sleep or who frequently wake with nightmares can be given a gentle and harmless tea made from one of these.
- *Lettuce* What an ambiguous remedy this is! A tea made with chopped lettuce leaves infused for 20 minutes in 1½ cups of boiling water is reputed to bring sleep and so is eating the leaves but lettuce is also considered to be a diuretic and by some to be an aphrodisiac. Maybe one drops exhausted by all the activities resulting from a night-time draught.

To Banish Nightmares

An infusion of betony was considered an appropriate night-time tea if you suffered from nightmares whilst the most popular nightcap to remedy this problem was made with valerian and I give two useful recipes which should not be taken regularly but only in an emergency.

- *Valerian tea I* Infuse ¼ teaspoon each of peppermint, lemon balm and vervain and 1 teaspoon of grated valerian root for 15 minutes in 1 cup of boiling water. Sweeten with honey.
- *Valerian tea II* Infuse ½ teaspoon each of grated nutmeg and grated valerian root in 600ml(1 pint) of boiling water.
- *Other useful teas* All the following can be used to prevent nightmares: camomile with a pinch of cinnamon and sweetened with honey; sage; hor-

se's tail; lady's mantle; anise; fennel and dill.

● *A digestive* Eating unsuitable or difficult-to-digest food (peanuts, cheese) late at night is one of the prime causes of nightmares. Here is another digestive for those who do not listen to good advice. Take the ground seeds from 1 cardamom pod, 2 drops of peppermint oil, 1 teaspoon of sugar and 1 pinch of bicarbonate of soda in 1 cup of boiling water.

SKIN DISORDERS AND IRRITATIONS

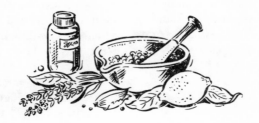

FAIR OF FACE

'The child that is born on the Sabbath day is blithe, bonny, good and gay' – but as far as I was concerned that child could be all of those things provided I was the one who was 'fair of face' for I took this to mean that if you had a good skin you could survive being plain and portly and actually come out on top. The ego becomes diminished when the skin is poor and even the most beautiful person feels less sure of themselves when they have a pimple upon the end of their nose. Most skin conditions, from a minor rash to acne, are brought about by a poor diet, allergic reaction, emotional upheaval, stress or hormonal imbalance and most of these issues have been covered elsewhere. However for those who have specific problems the following might help.

Old-fashioned Beauty Tips

- *Sallow skin* Rosemary flowers boiled in white wine will lighten sallow skin.

- *Wrinkles* A wash of lady's mantle or neat gin softens wrinkles. Apricot oil rubbed into the most sensitive, soft skin every night will also help.
- *Oily skin* This may benefit from a covering of mashed strawberries.
- *Hard, leathery patches of skin* These can be softened with pineapple juice or a mash of papaya. Both fruits contain enzymes which are used as meat tenderizers!
- *The morning dew* Whatever the problem you could always try the age old beauty tip of bathing the face in the morning dew.
- *Fenugreek seeds* A tea made from fenugreek seeds will purify the blood and make you look, smell and feel delightful.

BLACKHEADS

Blackheads are caused by the oil in the pores of the skin becoming trapped by grease or dirt. When this comes into contact with the air it turns black. Cleanse the skin regularly and thoroughly using a facial steamer and boiling water containing one or all of the following healing herbs: comfrey, peppermint, yarrow, thyme. This treatment softens and expands the pores after which it may be possible to expel the blackheads with the use of gentle pressure and scrupulously clean cotton wool. Follow this up with an astringent, healing face mask containing yoghurt or kaolin – several of the masks suggested for **Acne** will work very well, particularly the tomato paste mask.

FRECKLES

God-given and nowadays considered attractive, freckles were at one time thought to be a bane. They are caused by a melanin pigmentation in the skin and cannot be removed, only temporarily lightened. Herbal lotions made with elderflower, lime flowers, lady's mantle, the juices of cranberry and lemon or old-fashioned castor oil were all pressed into use as skin lighteners and these do actually work although another suggested concoctions of bitter almonds, brimstone and barley might give rise to a more pallid hue than expected. Alternatively you might try dabbing your face with the blood of a bull.

● *Horseradish and sour milk* Mix 4 tablespoons of sour milk with 1 tablespoon of ground oatmeal and 1 teaspoon of freshly grated horseradish. Apply the paste to the freckles taking great care to avoid the area around the eyes as the fumes can cause stinging. Leave for half an hour then wash off.
● *Pumpkin seeds* Pound to a paste with olive oil and use to keep skin soft and white and reduce freckles. The flesh of

pumpkin will also heal red patches and small burns.

BLEMISHES AND PIMPLES

These are temporary problems, the causes of which may vary from contact with a rough and bristly surface to an excess of alcohol or exposure to cold winds. Yoghurt will help to soothe sore patches as will marigold and wheat-germ oil.

● *The leaves of raspberry, strawberry or blackberry* Boil 50g(2oz) of the leaf gently in 1 litre(1¾ pints) of water for three minutes then infuse for a further five. This makes a very pleasant and soothing wash for itching skin especially if it is caused by small pimples or scabs.
● *Raspberry mask* Mix 25g(1oz) of mashed raspberries to a paste with 1 teaspoon each of plain yoghurt and finely ground oatmeal. Leave on the face for 10 minutes to clear minor blemishes.

SPOTS

One cause of these eruptions which we all know and love is using a face pack containing yeast. This will ultimately have a fine effect but may, within a few hours of applying it, stir up the skin rather too well.

● *Garlic* To kill spots instantly rub them with raw garlic.
● *Comfrey, honey and garlic* The following is a remedy for persistent pustules. Pound a handful of fresh comfrey leaves with enough honey to make a paste and for each tablespoon take 1 small well-mashed garlic clove. Mix them

together, apply on a small piece of warmed cabbage leaf and tie in place. Go to bed and do not open the door to anyone! It really does work and on quite nasty places.

• *A night-time ointment* Melt 25g(1oz) of beeswax in a bain-marie. Add 100g(4oz) of pure honey, stir until cool then pot. Seal tightly, keep in a cool place and apply to infected spots – it works best if the area is kept covered afterwards.

Wheatgerm and Honey Scrub
1 tablespoon wheatgerm
2 teaspoons clear honey
1 teaspoon sunflower oil
1 teaspoon fresh lemon juice

Mix all the ingredients together to make a thick paste and apply it in small circular rubbing movements to the face and neck. Leave for five minutes then wash off with warm water. Splash with cold before patting dry. Use once or twice a week. In between times avoid soap and wash your face in clear water only.

MINOR IRRITATIONS

Patches of itching skin for which you can find no identifiable answer may occur on any part of the body and many of the remedies suggested for **Measles** and **Eczema** will help. Oral antibiotics often create this problem and the very best antidote is to eat a large amount of plain live yoghurt. A large handful of oats or ground oatmeal thrown into a warm bath will ease all-over itches.

Many skin irritations can be caused by the soap you use so try the alternative of making your own with the herbs and essential oils that suit your skin best.

Herbal Soap
1 large block olive or vegetable oil soap
25g(1oz) finely chopped herbs
a few drops of essential oil
1 tablespoon finely ground oatmeal

Grate the soap into a basin and add the remaining ingredients. Heat gently in a bain-marie until they melt and mix well. Line an egg box with waxed paper and pour the soap into each section. It is better, of course, if you have the correct moulds for soap-making but this is a neat alternative.

• *Purple loosestrife lotion* Boil 100g (4oz) of dried purple loosestrife for five minutes in 1 litre(1¾ pints) of water then leave to stand for 10 minutes. Use as a compress to bring relief to areas of itching skin, whether caused by eczema, impetigo or guilt.

ACNE

Acne is a few or a collection of pimples and pustules which erupt over the face and back and is caused by the sebaceous glands, which are attached to each side of the hair follicle, overproducing and becoming blocked. Stress, poor diet, allergic reaction and hormonal imbalances occurring mostly during adolescence, and occasionally during the menopause in women and also prior to periods, may all create the conditions under which acne will erupt.

Contrary to popular belief greasy, dirty skin and hair do not cause acne but in order to prevent infection it is essential to maintain strict cleanliness externally and internally. Many sources advocate washing with pure soap and water but I believe that it is best to keep the face clean with warm water alone, using a small, slightly abrasive face sponge. I also believe strongly in the benefits of warm, healing face masks which will soften and cleanse the clogged pores without adding to the problem. It is when acne becomes infected by pressing and picking and thus allowing dirt to infiltrate the vulnerable areas that the major problems arise. Up until that point acne is just one of those aggravations which disappear after a while. I do not think that it is wise to use facial scrubs and peelers, heavy cleansing lotions and strong astringents, nor to try to cover the affected area with masking creams and powder. Fresh water, particularly sea water, fresh air and sunlight will do far more to improve the condition of the skin and so will looking to your diet and that euphemistic 'inner cleanliness'.

Diet

Cut out all fats and eat plenty of good greenstuff. An excellent breakfast time cocktail to be taken daily in times of crisis is a combination of beetroot, celery and tomato juice. When the condition has cleared reduce the dose to twice a week as a preventative. Blackstrap molasses taken daily is another essential as is honey or honey and lemon juice tea at night. Liquorice, either in a tea or as sweets, was the old-fashioned answer to spots and is considerably more palatable than cod liver oil and cold baths.

If you suffer frequently from these frustrating outbreaks try to pinpoint the times when they are most likely to occur and take evasive action beforehand by going on a three-day diet of grapes and water or fruit juice. However this should only be attempted when you are 'resting', otherwise you will become tired and even more stressed. Another

preventative tonic to be taken before a period (if this is the time when acne begins to make itself felt) is made by simmering 25g(1oz) of fresh sorrel in 1 litre(1¾ pints) of water for 10 minutes.

● *A decoction of horsetail (Equisetaceae)* Taken regularly this was considered to be the best possible tonic to cure acne and eczema. It also encourages the white spots on fingernails to disappear but I believe that this is because it improves the general state of health. Horsetail decoction also provides an excellent healing wash for most skin conditions.

Cleansing Lotions and Packs

● *Witch hazel* Use this either by itself or mixed with rose water or cider apple vinegar. A very old-fashioned remedy was to use it in equal quantities with cabbage juice.
● *Lemon juice* Either dab it on neat – which is especially valuable if you have been picking – or with an equal quantity of water to wash a larger area.
● *Thyme and lemon lotion* Boil several sprigs of fresh thyme in 2 cups of water for two minutes and leave to infuse for five. Strain and add the juice of ½ lemon. Use this to rinse the face at least twice a day.
● *Nettle tea* Use nettle tea to wash with and to drink. Parsley juice and the expressed juice of comfrey leaves are also invaluable lotions.
● *Herbal lotions* Lady's mantle, yarrow, marigold, lavender and camomile may all be useful as may any healing herbal vinegar diluted with water.
● *Soapwort* Wash with a soapwort solution if the skin is very greasy.
● *Camomile, lime, sage, thyme* Any one or a mixture of these herbs in a warm poultice will soothe and heal. Stand the

herbs in a bowl of boiling water until they have softened and cool a little before applying. Many people prefer to use them as a 'steamer' to open the pores but this may cause infection to spread.

• *Comfrey* Both the powdered root and the leaves make a healing poultice and an excellent lotion.

• *Lettuce leaves* Boiled and applied warm these help to soothe overheated skin. They also work wonders on sunburn.

• *Grape skins* If you are feeling extravagant a poultice of grape skins is said to be the very best method of healing acne.

• *Quince* The mucilaginous juice from simmered quince seeds will help damaged skin to heal.

• *Marigold and wheatgerm oil* Pound 2 tablespoons of fresh or 1 tablespoon of dried marigold petals with 4 tablespoons of warm wheatgerm oil (a good source of vitamin E). Strain into a little bottle and use to heal those small scars or blemishes caused by acne, burns and thread veins. Vitamin E oil will also work wonders.

Sulphur Mask
1 teaspoon sulphur powder
2 tablespoons fuller's earth
1 beaten egg white
bottled water

Mix the ingredients together using enough bottled water to make a smooth paste. Although this is an efficient deep-cleansing mask make an allergy test before using it because some skins may suffer an adverse reaction to sulphur. To do this spread a little of the mixture over the skin on the inside of the elbow. Leave for a few minutes then rinse off and pat dry. Check the skin for any reaction.

• *Plum mask* Mash 250g(8oz) of boiled plums with 1 teaspoon of almond oil to make a thick paste. Many acne sufferers also have the double problem of a dry skin and this mask, used cautiously, may help to alleviate it.

Tomato Paste Mask
4 good-sized tomatoes
finely ground oatmeal
1 teaspoon clear honey

Purée and sieve the tomatoes. Mix the ingredients to make a smooth paste and rub it gently over the skin, concentrating on the worst affected areas. Leave on the skin for 10 minutes then rinse off with warm water. This remedy is more of a preventative for it cleanses and clears blackheads and blocked pores like magic.

• *Yoghurt and oatmeal* Mix natural yoghurt and fine oatmeal to a thick paste, apply and leave to dry. This paste can be used as a basic mask to which you can add herb, fruit and vegetable extracts to suit your skin type and problem.

• *Potato mask* Make a thick paste with 1 tablespoon each of extracted potato juice and fuller's earth. Use as a deep-cleansing and healing mask for spotty skins.

Onion Mask
1 tablespoon onion juice (extracted in a blender)
1 tablespoon kaolin powder
1 teaspoon clear honey

Mix the ingredients together to form a thick paste and use on blemished, oily skins.

• *Essential oils of camomile, lavender and myrrh* These oils may all be dabbed neat on to badly affected areas and are particularly useful if you have dry skin, although essential oils do become absorbed so rapidly into the skin that you may need a second dab.

● *Calendula oil, cream and lotion* Use any of these alternatives to heal and nourish acneous skin which is very dry. It is a mistake to believe that only oily skins are prone to acne – people with dry skins have double trouble.

● *Aloe vera* Soaps and gels made from aloe vera purport to heal skin damaged by acne. The liquid obtained from the fleshy leaves certainly helps to soothe sunburn. It is probably worth trying as an alternative to the old-fashioned brimstone and lard treatment and it is certainly worth using an aloe vera shampoo if other types irritate your skin.

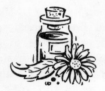

BOILS

Unless a boil is caused by an outside infection such as a splinter or picking with dirty fingers it is most probably the result of a poor state of health and can usually be taken as a pretty fair indicator that you need a change of either diet or scene. If you suffer from boils continuously you should take professional advice. Such advice many years ago would have comprised a blood purifier of black molasses or treacle and flowers of sulphur, hot compresses or 'cupping' – a process which it intrigues me to know is still carried out even today. The theory is that one takes a small-mouthed jar well rinsed in boil-

ing water and, as soon as is feasible without scalding the patient, places the mouth of the jar over the boil then waits for it to cool. Suction does the rest and provided the boil is at a stage ready for treatment the core will come out neatly and without unnecessary pain.

One of the most constantly recommended methods of 'drawing' a boil that I have come across is to take the skin of a hard-boiled egg – that is the thin membrane between white and shell – and wrap it over the boil. I am told this never fails to work. A madonna lily petal steeped in brandy and used rough side down will draw a boil to a head then when it has satisfactorily dispersed the smooth side should be used to heal it. Onions baked to a pulp and used in a poultice and leek, cabbage and rape treated in the same way or pounded with lard to make a healing unguent were all pressed into service, but I suspect that the problem might not have arisen if plenty of healthy green vegetables and foods rich in minerals and vitamins had been eaten in the first place.

When treating boils absolute cleanliness is essential for both your own sake and that of your patient. Make sure that your hands are well scrubbed in soap and water before and after dealing with it. Always use boiled water and sterile dressings and never, ever squeeze a boil for it is not only potentially dangerous but murderously painful. Hot compresses are the most sensible and safe method of bringing a boil to a head and giving relief from the pain.

There are a great many old-fashioned herbal remedies which I mention below but among the least complex and most satisfactory hot compresses are hot water or hot water and salt. Also recommended for both simplicity and efficacy is a solution of 1 tablespoon of Epsom salts and 1 teaspoon each of bicarbonate of soda and boric acid powder in 4 cups of boiling water. Use a soft compress of cotton wool which should be burned or flushed away as soon as it is discarded.

Although it is best to let a boil come to a head without covering, this is not always practical so cotton wool covered with lint and taped in place is the best alternative. Poultices can also be kept on, taped in place, until they have cooled.

Preventative Measures

If you are prone to boils take sulphur regularly.

Drink plenty of water and avoid fatty foods, chocolate and stimulants.

Sunshine and a daily swim in unpolluted sea water are the best although not always the most practical solutions. Investigate sensible alternatives.

A three to four day fast on fruit juices will cleanse and purify when you feel your system becoming clogged.

● *Honey* Equal quantities of honey, fresh lemon juice, fresh orange juice and cod liver oil mixed and taken three times a day is an excellent tonic when you are feeling tired and run down.
● *Iodine* Swab an incipient boil with iodine three times a day to stop it developing further. Paint around a boil with rubbing alcohol or iodine to bring it to a neat head and prevent infection.
● *Red clover, nettle and sassafras tea* This brew purifies the system.

Emergency Measures

● *Honey* Apply warm honey, honey and oil – wheatgerm for preference – or honey, fresh fig and thyme simmered together or dip half a fresh fig in honey and apply it cut side down.
● *Comfrey* Pulp the leaves with honey and garlic and apply.
● *Lemon* Apply half a lemon cut side down.
● *Wheatgerm and carrot* Grate a raw carrot into 1 tablespoon of wheatgerm oil. Apply as a thick poultice and leave over the boil.
● *Bread poultice* Soak bread in boiling water (you can add 1 good teaspoon of mustard powder if you like) until it is soft and apply still hot but not boiling as a poultice. This is a genuinely effective method of bringing a boil to a head.
● *Linseed poultice* Crush 1 good handful of fresh linseeds and add as much boiling water as you need to make a paste. Apply thickly and cover.
● *Fenugreek* Apply a poultice of crushed fenugreek seeds which have been boiled in water for 10 minutes.
● *Slippery elm and eucalyptus oil* Mix the powdered bark of slippery elm with eucalyptus oil to make a thick, soothing poultice that is also effective on cuts, whitlows and carbuncles.
● *Yarrow, dock, chickweed, catnip, burdock or wild pansy (hearts' ease)* The leaves of any of these herbs steamed and softened may be used as a drawing, healing poultice but do make sure that they come from a clean source. Sorrel cooked and reduced to a pulp is reputed to clear a boil overnight.
● *Essential oils of camomile, lavender, lemon, myrrh or thyme* Use either direct or on a hot compress to relieve pain and reduce infection.

- *Zinc* Take a daily course of zinc until the boil has healed.
- *Calendula extract* This is recommended as a safe and healing lotion.

ABSCESSES AND CARBUNCLES

An abscess is a very severe boil which usually requires professional treatment.

A carbuncle is a many-headed or collection of boils in one place and that place is usually the posterior. The best old-fashioned advice that I can conjure up is to sit in a bowl of hot water into which one of the solutions given for **Boils** has been stirred. Carbuncles in any other place may be treated as a severe boil and any of those remedies used, especially a thick poultice of slippery elm.

Kaolin poultice followed by a dressing of Golden Lion ointment applied on cotton wool and taped into place was the treatment for every type of infected pustule and it did seem to clear them up quickly and without too much agony. However it did not, I suspect, get to the source of the problem.

NETTLE RASH

Although commonly believed to be a reactionary rash caused by nettles, urticaria can actually be the result of an allergy towards almost anything (see **Allergies**). In its mildest form it is aggravating and irritating but it can be serious if the reaction is violent enough to cause those areas surrounding the lips and eyes to swell and if the soft membranes inside the throat and mouth swell enough to make suffocation imminent.

The most common reaction suffered by the majority of us is that which is caused by a cat scratch or insect bite and is instantly identifiable as a red weal which itches. Certain plants inflict the same kind of rash as a nettle sting and strong sunlight can have a similar effect. Rubbing well with the astringent leaves of dock relieves the discomfort of nettle stings but it is probably safer to dab any irritations with calamine lotion. Nettle tea, on the basis of fighting fire with fire, has been known to effect a cure.

PSORIASIS

This not uncommon condition can be identified by scaly, dry blotches most generally on the soft inner side of elbows, knees, crotch and occasionally scalp and forehead. They become rough and red with a silvery soft, scabby appearance. It is often considered to be an indication of poor health and hygiene which at one time had unfortunate connotations. Fair-skinned people seem to suffer from it more than dark-skinned and although it looks unpleasant it is not infectious and the victim should not be treated as a pariah. Psoriasis may be caused by using detergents and in some cases it is the result of an allergic reaction.

There was nothing mystical about the old-fashioned treatments for it which still hold good today. A diet of raw foods was recommended including whey milk for breakfast and slippery elm and honey at night. If the patient was of a nervous disposition either sage tea or golden rod tea were given to calm and strengthen. More up-to-date suggestions might include a vitamin A supplement, cod liver oil or evening primrose oil.

Drinks and Lotions

Burdock and Camomile Drink
25g(1oz) each dried burdock seed and
dried camomile flowers
600ml(1 pint) water
honey

Simmer the burdock seed and
camomile flowers in the water in a
covered pan for 15 minutes. Strain
through a clean cloth and sweeten to
taste with honey. Keep refrigerated.
Take 3 tablespoons four times daily for
two weeks. This will also strengthen the
body against irritations of the skin,
boils, styes and rheumatism.

● *Witch hazel, nettle extract or calendula
extract* Swab each affected area with
one of these lotions soaked into clean
cotton wool.
● *Wheatgerm oil and castor oil* Mix 1
teaspoon each of wheatgerm oil and
castor oil into 1 eggcup of sunflower oil.
Rub gently into the affected area.
● *Calendula* Add 2 drops of calendula
(marigold) oil and 1 drop of oregano oil
to 1 small cup of olive oil. Rub into the
area.
● *Marigold lotion for an irritated scalp*
Boil 4 marigold heads in 4 cups of water
for two minutes. Allow to cool then
massage this lotion well into the scalp.
Wash with a very mild shampoo or a
solution of soapwort. Add lemon juice
or cider vinegar to the rinsing water to
ensure a thorough rinse.

SHINGLES

Herpes zoster is the technical name for
this skin condition which is thought to
be related to chicken pox and which
appears to be brought on by extreme
tiredness, emotional tension and being
generally run down. It is an inflammation of the major sensory nerves and
therefore confines itself to 'quarters' of
the body but no description can
accurately conjure up the sheer pain
and irritation and the debilitating after-
effects. Shingles is very unpleasant and
requires professional advice at any time
but especially if it is on the face because
precautions must be taken to protect
the eyes. I have to take a somewhat
defeatist attitude and say that all one
can do about shingles is to try to relieve
the discomfort, and to this end I know
of many people who have used the
services of an acupuncturist as an alternative to the time-honoured aspirin and
calamine lotion. Many of the remedies
suggested under **Anxiety**, **Nervousness** and **Skin Disorders and Irritations** can be used to bring strength
and comfort.

Drink and Diet

The most useful remedies are those
which one might take for nervous disorders – vitamin B complex, a regular
bowl of oats, a fruit juice fast, a daily
tablespoon each of orange juice and
castor oil, and nettle, sage, camomile,
valerian or blackberry leaf tea.

Soothing Oils and Waters

The most comforting thing that I can
remember using when I had shingles on
my face was a cold compress which had
been soaked in tincture of hypericum
(St John's wort) and this was no mystical panacea but a very genuine relief.
Infusions of calendula, camomile,
horsetail and horehound can also be
used to soothe the affected area. Essential oil of rose in the bath water will
bring peace of mind and a hop pillow
may help you to sleep.

• *Lemon, geranium, camomile or lavender*
These soothing essential oils may be
diluted in a base oil and rubbed on to
the rash or alternatively into the soles of
the feet.
• *Mullein and mallow compress* Take
25g(1oz) each of dried mullein, mallow
roots and marsh mallow roots. Put
them to simmer for three minutes in 3
litres(5¼ pints) of water. Strain and use
on a compress throughout the day and
night to reduce heat and irritation.
• *Vitamin E oil* This will reduce the
pain and irritation of the rash and also
help to prevent scarring if shingles is on
the face.
• *Calendula or hypericum ointment* Both
ointments will soothe and heal.

External Ulcers

External ulcers are the result of a small
wound or insect bite which refuses to
heal. Varicose ulcers are those which
open on a varicose vein and I strongly
advise against anyone neglecting them
– seek a professional opinion.

Ulcers should be kept dry and protected. Simple remedies would have
included bathing with a herbal lotion
such as horsetail, marigold, sage, thyme,
rosemary, camomile or red clover, leaving the area to dry and then dressing
with comfrey ointment or the more
modern alternative of vitamin E oil
straight from a capsule. If the ulcerated
area is not severe many of the remedies
given for **Boils** may bring relief.

Warts and Verrucas

Both warts and verrucas are caused by
an infectious virus and are known as
verrucas when found on the soles of the
feet. Nobody really knows why warts

appear and nobody can foretell their
disappearance although many people
have made a living out of attempting
to do so. Even today there are wart
charmers still working and, to be fair,
most of them have an altruistic attitude
about their undoubted gift. However at
one time a pretty penny could be made
out of convincing the gullible public
that if they rubbed their warts in a piece
of rancid meat and thrust it beneath a
dung heap the warts would in time disappear – which of course they did but
more in the nature of things than due to
magic. You could if you chose (but I
don't advise it) prick each wart with a
new pin which would then be driven
into a tree after which the warts would
one by one drop off. A delightful model
of Medieval malevolence was the practice of rubbing the warts with a piece of
bark or meat which was then wrapped
enticingly in a small parcel and dropped conveniently for an unwary travel-
ler to pick up, the intention being that
he picked up your warts as well.

Old-fashioned Remedies

I have to say quite honestly that I do
not know whether the following
remedies, some of which I have tried,
do actually work or whether it was just
the passage of time that did the trick. I
will leave you to make up your own
minds. However it is always a good idea
to wear rubber shoes when visiting
swimming pools to guard against the
possibility of 'catching' a verruca.

• *Banana skin* Strap a small piece of
banana skin, soft side down, over the
wart and leave overnight. Do this for at
least one week. The soft side of a broad
bean pod or a piece of pineapple are
said to work equally well.
• *Celandine, dandelion, figwort, houseleek or*

fig stalk The juice of any of these, applied through a small piece of cardboard with a suitable sized hole cut in it will remove a wart if used for three days. This remedy also works on corns. The juice of celandine is so corrosive that it was at one time employed by beggars to induce blisters on their bodies and thereby raise sympathy.

- *Lemon or vinegar* The pure juice of a lemon or vinegar in which the rinds of 2 lemons have been macerated is a simple alternative to the previous remedy.
- *Garlic* You can rub your wart with garlic – of course!
- *Onion* Cut an onion in half. Scoop out the centre of one half and fill the cavity with coarse sea salt. Allow this to dissolve and use the resulting liquid on the wart as often as possible.

A Healthy Head
of Hair

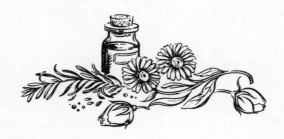

Hair is not just an attractive frame to the face, an adjunct to our vanity to be teased into a fashionable style which makes a statement about ourselves. It is indeed our crowning glory, a symbol of our virility, our desirability, and when it starts to fall out or turn grey our morale takes a decided turn for the worse. Such is our state of mind on the subject that remedies for baldness litter the pages of old encyclopedias and as little as 50 years ago otherwise sensible and seemly matrons would cheerfully pour a mixture of sulphate of iron and red wine over their heads to prevent greying. Nowadays we do far worse but would do better by ensuring that our hair is kept healthy and in a good condition by maintaining a sensible diet and lifestyle and trying to avoid using harsh and possibly damaging products on our hair.

It was thought that prematurely greying hair was caused by a diet deficient in copper and iron and could be halted by a greater intake of prunes, radishes, onions, lentils, raspberries and rye bread, but gipsy women with a thick mane of glossy black hair would swear that drinking nettle tea had the same effect. In Italy women macerated the rind taken from several green oranges in olive oil for two months and massaged this into their hair to restore the colour when it had faded. In an age when there were few artificial aids to hair beauty, women grew their hair until it reached their toes. The other side of that coin is that we may now view baldness as a sign of extreme virility or why else would all these strapping chaps shave their heads?

Natural Solutions

Bay rum, which was made from the leaves of the bayberry tree, was a very popular hair tonic with both men and women.

Another remedy for darkening grey

hair was to make 600ml(1 pint) of strong Indian tea using 25g(1oz) of leaf and let it stand until cold. The tea was then strained and mixed with 100ml(4 fl oz) of Jamaica rum and applied once a day.

Soapwort and Camomile Shampoo
1 tablespoon each dried camomile
flowers and powdered soapwort root
275ml(½ pint) boiling water

Infuse the herbs in the water overnight then strain before using. Soapwort – any part of the herb – makes a soapy liquid which whilst it does not lather will thoroughly cleanse the hair. Camomile will strengthen and lighten weak hair but other herbs may be used to meet specific problems.

An Excellent Hair Tonic
100g(4oz) each nettle leaves,
nasturtium flowers, seeds and leaves
and box leaves
600ml(1 pint) rum

Chop the leaves and put them in a glass jar with the rum to macerate for three weeks. Strain through a fine nylon sieve pressing well to extract all the liquid. Massage frequently into the scalp to condition the hair. It is perhaps best to do this at night.

Home-made Brilliantine
50g(2oz) white wax
400ml(12 fl oz) olive oil
4 drops each bergamot and clove oil
2 drops geranium oil

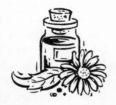

Melt the wax in a bowl over hot water then beat in the warm olive oil followed by the essential oils. Remove from the heat and continue beating until cooling. Pour into pots and seal when cold. Apply a little on the fingertips and smooth through the hair to give gloss and condition.

● *Beer* Rinse the hair with beer to give body.
● *Lemon juice* Comb lemon juice through the hair and leave to dry naturally to give light streaking – if you can dry the hair in the sun the effect can be quite startling. It works best on light brown hair.
● *To lighten hair* Dye with rhubarb root or stem. Rinse with camomile, elderflower or mullein.
● *To give red hues* Rinse with saffron, ginger root, marigold or red oak bark. Use red henna to dye the hair.
● *To highlight dark hair* Rinse with cloves, lemon verbena or box.
● *To colour dark, greying hair* Rinse with rosemary, sage or walnut leaves and shell.

DANDRUFF

Dandruff is a scaly condition of the scalp caused by the hair follicle becoming blocked with excess sebum and is therefore associated with oily skin and acne. It can equally well be caused by stress and anxiety or by keeping the head covered.

Follow this routine. Wash the hair every other day using a mild baby shampoo then rinse the scalp in either warm water to which you have added 1 tablespoon of cider vinegar or a strong infusion of one of the following: burdock root, stinging nettles, raspberry leaves, sage, goosegrass, marjoram, parsley, quince seeds, rosemary or southern-wood. Any of the herbs can be added to soapwort shampoo.

Follow a diet high in fresh fruits, vegetables and protein.

- *Apple juice tonic* Mix together 1 tablespoon of pure apple juice and 3 tablespoons of warm water and massage into the scalp three times a week.
- *Rosemary and borax* Mix 5 tablespoons of strong rosemary infusion with a pinch of borax and massage into the scalp daily.
- *Nasturtium tea* Make a strong infusion with 1 drop of essential oil of thyme added to it. Use to rinse the hair or massage the scalp.

ITCHY SCALP

True eczema is a condition which you will already know yourself to be vulnerable to and have identified. However an itchy scalp can be caused by inadequate rinsing after shampooing, covering the head, chlorine, salt, chemicals in hair preparations, central heating or an allergic reaction. It is best overcome by using a mild vinegar rinse before shampooing and to shampoo every other day with a very mild shampoo followed by a herbal, lemon or vinegar rinse. Use a scalp conditioner regularly. Catmint, comfrey, nettle (especially dead white nettle), parsley, raspberry leaves, quince, rosemary, southern-wood, thyme and yarrow are healing and soothing and will improve the condition of the hair. Essential oils of lavender and juniper will also help. See as well the lavender oil for **Eczema** – not only is it an excellent oil to use for this condition but many other herbal oils can be made in the same way. One or 2 drops of bergamot oil added to an eggcup of sunflower oil is another heal-ing unguent, and olive oil heated with rosemary, nettle or catnip alleviates an itchy scalp.

- *Witch hazel* Used by itself or mixed with a flower or herbal infusion, especially yarrow and thyme, witch hazel is an excellent method of cleaning oily hair when the scalp is itching.
- *Egg and orange shampoo* Whisk 1 egg and 1 tablespoon of orange juice into 300ml($\frac{1}{2}$ pint) of warm soapwort infusion. Massage the mixture well into the hair and leave for 10 minutes. Rinse thoroughly with luke warm water. This is a super remedy for oily hair and an itchy scalp.

DRY, THINNING HAIR AND HAIR LOSS

Hair loss can be caused by anxiety, tension, shock, drugs, illness or hormonal upheavals including pregnancy. When the hair comes out in patches it is known as alopecia. Drink lots of water and improve the diet by supplementing it with brewer's yeast and, according to some sources, beetroot juice. It is also thought that a silica deficiency might cause falling hair. Use a very mild or herbal shampoo daily and a protein or oil-based conditioner. Massaging the scalp regularly with a restorative oil or tonic will also promote growth. Treat the hair carefully using only a very soft brush or, preferably, a wide-toothed comb. If the condition does not improve consult a specialist.

Old-fashioned cures included steeping a sliced onion in rum for hours and using the resulting liquid as a massage which, although it works very efficiently to halt falling hair, is a little antisocial. Other remedies incorporated chilli, garlic and castor oil. More practical infusions may be made from mallow root, parsley seed, catmint, rosemary, marjoram and nasturtium.

• *Hot oil conditioner* Heat a small bowl of olive oil or a herbal oil and massage it well into the scalp until the hair is completely saturated. Comb through with a wide-toothed comb then massage again. Cover your hair in a plastic cap and swathe your head in a hot towel. Leave overnight for the best results and shampoo in the morning with a mild baby shampoo.

• *Essential oils of cedarwood and southernwood* Dilute 3 drops of each oil in 1 teaspoon of base oil and massage into the scalp for hair loss and alopecia.

• *Eucalyptus oil B.P.* Three parts of eucalyptus oil mixed with 1 part of clove oil rubbed into the scalp at night will prevent hair loss.

• *Yoghurt* Yoghurt alone, rubbed well into the scalp after shampooing and left for 10 minutes, will condition hair and clear up problems affecting the scalp but with 1 egg whisked into it it becomes doubly effective for fine, light and uncontrollable hair. Rinse well after using.

• *Southernwood tonic* Pour 5 tablespoons each of strong southernwood infusion and mild eau de Cologne into a bottle and shake well. Use diluted – 1 tablespoon of tonic to one of warm water – and massage into the scalp twice a week. Use only on oily hair which is showing signs of coming out but remember that a certain amount of hair loss is normal.

• *Rosemary and castor oil* Mix in the proportions of 2 tablespoons of castor oil to 4 drops of essential oil of rosemary. Massage the warmed oils into the hair, cover and leave overnight. Wash the next day using a mild shampoo. This is a healing conditioner to prevent hair loss after illness.

• *Watercress* Macerate 100g(4oz) of watercress in 100ml(4 fl oz) of alcohol for one week with 1 teaspoon of oil of geranium. Used as a tonic this promotes hair growth.

BALDNESS

I give below a range of remedies which have not as yet turned me into a millionaire. Many unscrupulous people have made their fortunes from the belief that baldness is a sign of 'sans eyes, sans teeth, sans everything' which nowadays is known to be patently untrue. However I glean quiet satisfaction from the thought that as women have until recently suffered the most obvious signs of ageing it is nice to know that something drops off the chaps so publicly.

The 'silly season' of remedies includes horseradish up each nostril, the thin rind of lemon applied to the temples or cow dung tied on to the head with a clean cloth which apparently only works with women: methinks there is a chauvinist at work.

• *Sunlight* As keeping the head covered is said to cause hair loss, exposing the head to the elements, within reason, is commonsense.

• *Nettles* Drink nettle tea to prevent hair loss. Rub nettle juice into the scalp. Nettle leaves and burdock root macerated in rum is another good hair restorer, as is nettle leaves macerated in warm vinegar. Another nettle remedy and one which was guaranteed to work was to macerate 50g(2oz) each of nettle tops and flowering tips of marjoram in 1 litre(1¾ pints) of brandy or rum for three weeks.

● *Onions* Rub the head with onion juice night and morning until red then anoint with honey. I have heard that one must suffer to be beautiful!

Garlic Hair Unguent
100g(4oz) fresh garlic
100g(4oz) beeswax
100g(4oz) honey

Crush the garlic very well and place it in a bowl with the beeswax. Stand this in a pan of hot water and heat until the wax has melted then add the honey and continue to heat, stirring well, until the mixture is hot. Remove from the heat and beat until cool. Put into pots and seal. Rub a little into the head each night.

● *Lavender or thyme* Either of these macerated in alcohol will restore hair if applied several times a week. A strong decoction will also prevent and arrest hair loss.
● *Rosemary* Apply either the essential oil or spirits of rosemary. However you could just wash with rosemary water and dry with a flannel.
● *Maidenhair and willow* Simmer a handful each of chopped maidenhair and willow leaves in olive oil. Add a pinch of cinnamon and remove from the heat. Leave to stand overnight then strain and apply nightly. Massage with olive oil as an easy alternative.
● *Beetroot juice* Drink this decoction rather than anoint the head with it.

CRADLE CAP

This is a scurfy patch on a new baby's head, usually at the front of the scalp, which looks dingy and oily. Some silly old women, as opposed to sensible old wives, worry new young mothers terribly with tales of poor hair growth and scalp infections. My own daughter was born with cradle cap which persisted for quite a long time but I am pleased to say that now, in her early teens, she has a magnificently luxurious and strong growth of hair. However it is important to wash and dry the scalp properly when the baby is bathed and it helps if you gently rub a little baby oil or sweet almond oil into the patch. It does ultimately disappear so do not worry unduly.

HEAD LICE

Every now and then panic-stricken notices will be sent from school indicating that head lice are once again proving a pest. These are tiny little parasites which suck blood from the skin and live in the hair. They irritate and they spread like fury in schools. They are most likely to have first occurred in an unhygienic home where children are neglected and were obviously far more prevalent 50 years ago than today. However with the fashion for long hair which is sometimes never untied or brushed the problem today may go unnoticed until it becomes a scourge. At one time every school in Britain was regularly visited by the 'nit' nurse who would shave the poor victim's head, but now the school will insist that you all buy and use a special shampoo and they will also instruct the children on the personal hygiene of never sharing head gear, brushes or combs and the necessity of washing and combing the hair regularly.

If your child does have head lice and you have an aversion to the recommended shampoo try instead washing the hair with cider vinegar which should be left on for half an hour before rinsing. This must be done several times a day to remove the lice and eggs. As a precaution against harbouring lice rinse the hair with a strong infusion of southernwood after shampooing.

Taking Care of the Hands and Feet

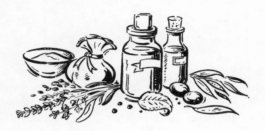

Cleansing and Pampering

Whilst we all view our faces every day with whatever degree of satisfaction our vanity leads us to and whilst our bodies usually make their ailments well and truly felt, we take our poor old hands and feet for granted and not until they are damaged do we realize how debilitating a mishap to them can be. They are the constant workhorses of the body. Many of our nastiest, niggling aches and pains stem from neglect of our feet and the inability to perform the most simple tasks can result from damaging our hands, so pampering and pandering to them is not vanity or self-indulgence but necessity.

Massage hands and feet every night and work out a routine of flexing and strengthening exercises which is a pleasantly therapeutic practice before going to bed. Keep nails well manicured and cared for and visit a chiropodist if any problems arise with the feet. Do not wear high heels all the time – most back aches and a lot of headaches are caused by ill-fitting fashion shoes. Change footwear several times daily and allow the feet as much freedom as possible. See also **Smelly Feet**.

Handy Hints

- *Hand cleanser* Wash dirty hands with oil and sugar. If you have been gardening oil and salt is better as it will also help to heal small cuts. Just wring and rub hands together with the mixture then wash off with warm water and dry on kitchen paper.
- *Honey* Warm honey, rubbed into the rough skin on elbows and knees is an effective remedy, as is the following recipe which also uses honey.

Honey Lotion
2 tablespoons clear honey
2 tablespoons almond oil
5 tablespoons rose water
1 tablespoon cider vinegar

Warm the honey in a bain-marie then beat in the almond oil. Warm the rose water and vinegar to the same temperature and beat them slowly into the honey mixture a little at a time. Continue beating until the mixture cools. Bottle and seal. This is a pleasant, soothing treatment for rough, dry hands.

Honey Paste for Cleansing
1 tablespoon clear honey
1 egg white
1 teaspoon glycerine
finely ground oatmeal

Mix together the honey, egg white and glycerine with enough oatmeal to make a paste and apply on areas of dry skin which have become dirty and discoloured such as knees, elbows, heels and hands. Leave for 30 minutes before bathing. This is an excellent method of cleaning the skin without scrubbing and causing damage.

Wheatgerm and Lanolin Cream
2 tablespoons anhydrous lanolin
1 tablespoon wheatgerm oil
1 teaspoon purified water, warmed

Melt the lanolin in a bowl over boiling water then stir in the wheatgerm oil followed by the warmed water. Remove the bowl from the heat and continue beating until the mixture is cool. Pot and seal. This is an excellent though sticky night cream for rough, sore hands.

Best Foot Forward

The best feet will always be those which have enjoyed the luxury of a footbath when they ache. One tablespoon of sea salt or household soda to a basin of warm water is very soothing whilst substituting 1 teaspoon of mustard powder warms and revives in cold weather. There are many footbaths mentioned in this book which will all bring considerable comfort but one of the best is a basin of strong nettle infusion with 1 tablespoon of cider vinegar added. This is absolute bliss but do not think too hard about the colour of your feet.

An Astringent Foot Freshener
¼ cup each rose water, witch hazel and distilled water
1 tablespoon spirits of camphor B.P.
a pinch of alum

Put all the ingredients into a large bottle and shake well. Use on a wad of cotton wool to cool and harden up hot, tired feet. Cucumber juice will also cool aching feet, especially in the summer, but it can irritate.

● *Yoghurt* Mix together 150ml(¼ pint) of natural yoghurt and 1 teaspoon of vinegar. Brush all over the feet to whiten discoloured skin and heal sore, hard patches. Leave for five minutes then rinse off.
● *Orris and oatmeal powder* Mix together 8 tablespoons of very finely ground oatmeal and 2 tablespoons of orris root powder. Pass them through a fine sieve. Keep in a tightly sealed pot and use inside rubber gloves and Wellington boots to prevent excess perspiration.
● *Olive oil massage cream* Melt together 2 tablespoons each of olive oil and

anhydrous lanolin in a bain-marie. Remove from the heat and beat constantly until the mixture cools. Pot and seal. Use nightly to alleviate dry and flaking skin on hands, feet, arms and legs.

BLISTERS

There cannot be one amongst us who has not at some time or another suffered from a blister, that nasty little bubble of tight skin under which fluid gathers and which is the inevitable result of constantly rubbing the sensitive tissue. The most common places for most of us to raise blisters are on the feet when we are breaking in new shoes or on hands and feet when we have been participating in some form of unaccustomed work or leisure. Although it is a great temptation to prick the bubble to release the liquid it is safer to cover the area with a medicated plaster which will bring relief from pressure and ensure that the blister does not become infected. Old-fashioned healers included cabbage leaves cooked in milk or a poultice of freshly grated carrot which, if you happen to be out of plasters, might be better than nothing. I think however that most of us would draw the line at rubbing the affected place with a live slug although the slimy trail exuded by these creatures does harden on contact with the air and in bygone days might well have been the only solution.

Novice workers on the land and at sea ensured that they hardened their hands and feet before they were put to unaccustomed labours by applying a mixture of spirits and tallow daily. A good rubbing with methylated or surgical spirit will have much the same effect. Woodcutters and farmers in some parts of Europe used a solution

made from boiled walnut husks to toughen their hands, but it also stains the skin so effectively that it was the dye once commonly used to counterfeit a swarthy complexion.

The antiseptic juice from garlic or garlic ointment was and may still be used to ensure healing whilst comfrey ointment remains a safe standby in the medicine cabinet. A paste of cornflour or cornflour and honey will prevent infection if the blister is broken. Large broken blisters which cannot be protected easily with a plaster should be dressed with boracic powder and covered with lint. Not only is this a useful piece of old-fashioned first aid but it is also handy if you happen to be allergic to plasters. It is an improvement on the ancient dressing of brimstone and sweet oil.

CORNS AND CALLOUSES

A succinct summary of corns taken from an Edwardian guide to healthy and wholesome womanhood states that they are small, hard, painful patches of skin on the feet and are the result of vanity. Although this seems heartless it is nevertheless true that the majority of lumps and bumps which we have on our feet are primarily caused by ill-fitting shoes. However callouses on the hands are more often caused by continuous manual work.

Both corns and callouses are the result of persistent rubbing and pressure on the skin. The old-fashioned method of removing rough, hard skin from feet, hands, elbows and knees was to rub gently with a pumice stone (a light-weight grey volcanic stone still available at most chemists), and I am sure that many of us will remember seeing our fathers rubbing calloused areas on fingers and hands with the abrasive strip on a box of Swan Vesta matches. Many people take great delight in cutting their own corns and some masochists advocated drawing a needle of worsted thread through the corn, cutting the thread at either end and leaving it there until the skin dropped off, both of which practices I view with horror as infections caused by over enthusiastic digging can create far-reaching problems. However if it is going to be done one should know that cutting corns at the time of the waning moon will ensure that they disappear forever! Better advice by far was to run barefoot in the early morning dew – in fact going barefoot as much as possible is good advice at any time.

Pleasing Preventatives

• *Soap and water* Wash the feet daily with soap and warm water, rubbing well between the toes. Dry well and dust with unscented baby powder. Not only will this prevent those really unpleasant soft corns between the toes but if you are already suffering from corns it will render them less painful.
• *Cloves* Five drops of clove oil in 5 tablespoons of sesame oil relieves aching feet and soothes sore areas.
• *Castor oil* Massage the feet daily with castor oil which acts as both prevention and cure. A mixture of castor oil and turpentine was used very frequently to harden the feet and hands and make them less susceptible to corns and callouses. If these already exist use a pumice stone after massaging to remove the hard skin.
• *Epsom salts and borax* Fill a bowl with warm water and add 2 tablespoons of Epsom salts and 1 tablespoon of borax. Soak the feet until the water is cold then dry thoroughly and massage

with witch hazel. This will soothe and harden the skin.
• *Oil and vinegar* Soak the feet well in a basin of warm water in which you have dissolved 2 tablespoons of bicarbonate of soda. Dry well and massage with a mixture of 3 tablespoons of sunflower oil and 2 teaspoons of cider vinegar.
• *Vinegar and water* This is an old-fashioned footbath which is very effective. So is either sea salt (4 tablespoons) or household soda (1 tablespoon) added to a large basin of warm water.
• *Massage* Massaging the feet every day is one of the most certain ways of alleviating and preventing problems. It is also the most extraordinarily therapeutic form of self-help in which you can indulge. The following cream is soothing, emollient and deodorizing.

Lavender Foot Cream
6 tablespoons anhydrous lanolin
3 tablespoons almond oil
3 tablespoons glycerine
2 drops essential oil of lavender

Melt the lanolin in a bowl standing in a saucepan of hot water. Warm the oil and glycerine in the same way then beat them both into the lanolin together. Continue beating until the mixture has emulsified and is nearly cool. Add the lavender oil then pot and seal. If you persistently suffer from chilblains substitute essential oil of geranium for the lavender.

Plasters and Poultices

• *Lemon* A poultice of lemon peel applied soft side down and left overnight will dispel corns whilst less stubborn hard skin should be painted twice daily with lemon juice.
• *Raw tomato or fresh pineapple* Either

of these will soften corns if bandaged against them.

● *Dandelion, celandine, sedum or marigold* The sap or juice from the crushed leaves of any of these plants if applied morning and night and left to dry will remove corns, callouses and soft warts. Ivy leaves soaked in vinegar was another well-recommended plant poultice.

● *Leeks* Soak leeks in water or vinegar for 24 hours and use as a poultice.

● *Onions* Apply either soft soap and roasted onion or a poultice of onions baked in the oven. Rape baked in the same way and used as a warm poultice was believed to be able to reduce pain and swelling from corns, chilblains, bunions, whitlows, boils, ear-ache and toothache!

● *Lilies* Whilst the petals of the lovely madonna lily, soaked in brandy and applied rough side down were frequently used to 'draw' whitlows and boils, the crushed bulb of the plant was used to dispel corns. The baked bulb was also utilized as a poultice for both whitlows and chilblains.

● *Garlic* Rub corns with garlic or garlic juice and cover with a thin slice of garlic. Leave it tied on overnight.

● *Oil of turpentine* Soak the feet well in a basin of hot water and ½ cup of Epsom salts or bicarbonate of soda to soften them up ready for treatment with turpentine, which should be painted on nightly and bandaged.

Balm for Corns
50g(2oz) coconut oil or lard
30ml(1 fl oz) oil of camphor
(camphorated oil)
15ml(½ fl oz) oil of turpentine

Melt the oil or fat in a bowl over boiling water then beat in the remaining ingredients. Continue beating until the mixture cools. Pot and seal. Rub corns with this balm day and night. This remedy is a sight safer than the unpleasant alternative that I came across which consists of boiling up nightshade berries with hog lard.

● *Tincture of iodine* Paint corns nightly with iodine to soften and disperse them.

● *Swede* Hollow out a swede and pack it with coarse salt. Leave to stand for 24 hours then use the resulting liquid to bathe corns night and morning.

● *Corn plasters* No matter how many modern marvels may be discovered countrymen will still swear by unwashed sheep's wool.

WHITLOWS

A whitlow is a painful infection around the cuticle of the fingernail. It rises from the base of the nail and forms a blister filled with matter and the top joint and tip of the finger become red and swollen. Whitlows are frequently considered to be an indication of a debilitated state of health usually clearing up with time and treatment, but in unusual circumstances they may be a chronic or long-term condition due to a dietary deficiency.

Take care of your hands when gardening and doing housework by wearing gloves and always washing dirty hands very well, drying them thoroughly and gently pushing the cuticles back to ensure that they do not become broken or torn. Never use cuticle clippers.

Whitlows must have been a fairly common nuisance in past times for the old books abound with remedies. Most of these rely upon the use of warm poultices and fomentations. The most practical and sensible is a kaolin poultice which is doubly effective if a splinter is the cause of the infection but I do stress that it should be applied warm and not piping hot! Another effective but somewhat callous cure was to cut a hole in a lemon which was then packed with salt and the offending digit thrust within. It is not surprising therefore that the alternatives of the white parts of boiled leeks mixed with lard or well-soaked comfrey leaves consistently found more favour.

Prevention is Better than Cure

Most whitlows arise from damaged cuticles and the following creams and hand bath will help strengthen and protect those vulnerable areas.

• *Lanolin and iodine nail strengthener* Melt 1 tablespoon of anhydrous lanolin in a bain-marie. Stir in ½ teaspoon of iodine, ensuring that it is properly mixed, then pour into a small pot. Seal when cold. Rub into the cuticles at night and leave on.
• *Cuticle softener* Mix together 1 tablespoonful each of castor oil and glycerine and use to massage the cuticles. Rinse off with warm soapy water then dry well and apply a hand cream (see page 177).
• *Lemon and iodine lotion* Biting one's nails and thus creating 'hang nails' is another silly thing to do and increases the danger of infection. Youngsters taking exams frequently suffer from whitlows not only because they become physically below par but because they chew their fingernails down to the quick. Mix together 2 teaspoons each of iodine and lemon juice and paint the nails daily with this unpleasant-tasting deterrent.
• *Olive oil hand bath* Steep the hands once a week in a bowl of warm olive oil

which not only softens the cuticles but improves the condition of the skin.

ATHLETE'S FOOT

Athlete's foot is a thoroughly unpleasant little fungus which relishes and thrives in the atmosphere created in changing rooms and swimming pools especially when the users of those facilities wear synthetic socks and shoes and never bother to dry their feet properly. It creates nasty, spongy little patches between the toes, particularly the fourth and fifth, which become extremely irritated and sore. The most simplistic answer is to ensure that the feet are always washed and dried well after any activity which causes damp or perspiration and that the area between the toes is dusted with an unscented talcum or a mixture of talcum and borax. Always change into dry socks and shoes and whenever possible wear natural absorbent fibres on the feet or porous insoles in shoes. In the summer it is not too difficult to wear open sandals but every effort should be made to allow as much air to the feet as possible even during the winter months.

Old-fashioned Answers

Wash the feet, especially between the toes, with warm soapy water. Dry scrupulously and dust well with powdered alum or flowers of sulphur. At one time a piece of lamb's wool saturated with garlic oil would have been inserted between the offending toes and rubbing with a little garlic oil is still a good idea, though a trifle smelly.

• *Vinegar* Wash with an equal quantity of cider vinegar and warm

181

water or cider vinegar and surgical spirit. Both lavender or rosemary vinegar can be used instead.

● *Goldenseal root or agrimony* Wash with a strong infusion of either.

● *Yoghurt* Massage well between the toes with natural live yoghurt and leave overnight, washing well in the morning and drying and dusting with an antifungal powder.

● *Thyme or rosemary* Add a few drops of the essential oil of either herb to an eggcupful of olive oil and rub assiduously into the affected area.

BUNIONS

Commonly believed by many people to be neither more nor less than another type of corn, bunions are instead a condition more akin to bursitis. Although some relief may be obtained by painting them with the remedies given under **Chilblains** and **Corns**, more sensible precautions are to ensure that footwear fits properly and pay a visit to a chiropodist.

If you do work which entails your standing for many hours wear good sensible shoes. Always ensure that children's footwear is accurately fitted by specialists for this is where the problems start.

CHAPS

In these modern labour-saving days when women no longer have to launder by hand then scurry out into a windy garden to peg the washing on the line the likelihood of suffering from chaps is more remote than it once was, for the unpleasantly red rough skin, sometimes with deep splits on fingers and knuckles, is a problem predominantly caused by subjecting your hands to very hot and cold water and leaving them damp, by using harsh detergents and also by exposure to cold wind. The old-fashioned way of taking care of hands after wet work was to rinse them in a borax solution and to dust them with oatmeal powder. However the commonsense approach must now be to wear gloves when undertaking household chores. One lady I know who has kept sheep for years stores a few pieces of unwashed fleece by the side of her sink and after drying her hands rubs them thoroughly with this oily wool which is rich in natural lanolin. Another countrywoman favours rubbing her hands with grease (once goose grease but now she uses lard) before rinsing them with elderflower water and patting them dry.

To Prevent and Cure

● *Lard* Because it was the most easily available unguent, lard was pressed into service to make the most unusual yet effective barrier creams. The blossoms of broom, gorse, marsh mallow and elderflower were left to simmer in a good quantity for some considerable time on the back of the kitchen range then strained and potted for everyday use. The method is very simple and can still be used as a cheap and easy alternative to commercial products. Into a pan of clarified lard or goose grease pack as many of the blossoms of your choice as it will take. Leave overnight in a warm place. The next day melt the fat again and strain it through a fine sieve, pressing well. Add more blossoms to the lard and repeat the process until the unguent takes on the colour of the blooms and smells rather more of flowers than of fat. Gorse blossoms produce the most gorgeous deep yellow result but the drawback is in collecting them for unless you wear stout gloves your hands will be in a worse condition than housework ever caused.

Elderflower Hand Lotion
4 tablespoons elderflower water
4 tablespoons glycerine
2 tablespoons witch hazel
1 tablespoon almond oil
1 tablespoon eau de Cologne
½ teaspoon borax

Put all the ingredients into a screwtop jar and shake well. Seal tightly and shake before using every time you wash your hands.

Rosemary Jelly
8 tablespoons rosemary water
1 tablespoon glycerine
2 teaspoons arrowroot

Warm the rosemary water and the glycerine in two separate bowls standing in pans of hot water. Stir the arrowroot into the glycerine to make a smooth paste then add the rosemary water. Continue to heat over simmering water, stirring continuously, until the mixture becomes jellified and transparent then pot. Seal when cold and keep refrigerated. This non-sticky hand cream can also be made with either orange flower or elderflower water instead of the rosemary water. It is very economical and very effective.

● *Milk* Soak the hands nightly in a bath of warm milk.

● *Wheatgerm oil* Massage with wheatgerm oil and cover with cotton gloves at night to heal sore, splitting hands.

CHILBLAINS

Chilblains, those painful and irritating areas of swollen flesh which surround the tips and joints of hands and feet and which change from livid white to lurid red when pressed, are one of the most debilitating yet common ailments to afflict the peoples of northern climates. The most probable reasons for them are diet and circulation but they are also caused by extreme changes of temperature and severe cold. There are many old-fashioned and simple remedies based upon either rubbing the area regularly with a healing cream or bathing it in a warm solution (although this may have been taken too far in the serious suggestion that one bathed one's feet in the chamber pot each morning). However these methods are effective not only because of the therapeutic values of the plants used but through the gentle warmth and massage which increases and stimulates circulation.

Evasive Action

To prevent chilblains from occurring keep the hands and feet as warm as possible but never hold them in front of direct heat when they are cold. Thaw out frozen hands or feet under gently running cold, not hot, water.

Investigate your diet for a deficiency in calcium and silicon – raw cabbage, spinach, lettuce, strawberries, lemons, oranges, figs, carrots, barley, oats, cheese, milk and yoghurt will all improve this deficiency and so will a vitamin B supplement – and ensure that both hands and feet are massaged daily throughout the year (particularly during those winter months when they are at their most vulnerable). I can vividly remember my grandmother sitting pinching the ends of her fingers, an exercise which I looked upon as nervous until she told me that it brought the blood to the end of the fingers, encouraged strong, pink fingernails and prevented chilblains.

Use plain oil or one of the creams suggested below to rub extremities already suffering from chilblains. Wear open shoes around the house or long knitted slippersocks which are a modern update on the flannel or chamois socks that were at one time in some countries standard winter clothing. Try not to wear synthetic shoes or Wellington boots for too long.

● *Massage* Make a routine of massaging the hands and feet morning and night throughout the year thus ensuring that the circulation is improved. Some people advocate massaging with salt and others with a tincture of bryony berries in gin but I believe that it is enough to use a good-quality vegetable oil with a few drops of essential oil of lavender or lemon added to it.

● *Hardening the feet and hands* Gipsy folk would have sworn that walking barefoot in the dew will prevent chilblains or that washing feet and hands morning and night in alternate bowls of hot and cold water insures against suffering. The remedies that I have suggested for hardening the hands and feet under **Blisters** and **Corns and Callouses** will also help to prevent the onset of chilblains as will rubbing vulnerable areas with the used halves of lemons which might otherwise be discarded (this will also whiten and improve the condition of the skin).

Painting the toes and fingers with nettle juice is another old country remedy but I think that a daily cup of nettle tea might do more to improve the circulation.

Relieving the Agony Immediately

● *A word of warning* Do not rub juices, liniments or harsh and abrasive substances on to broken chilblains. Use only the gentlest creams.

● *Onion* Rub the irritating digits with onion juice. A gentle poultice of onion boiled in water and placed on the chilblains nightly also has its champions and many sources advocate onion juice as a preventative as well as a cure.

● *Garlic* Rub chilblains with fresh garlic juice to reduce itching. Take garlic regularly to improve your health.

● *Friar's balsam* Put the feet in a bowl of gently warm water to which a good teaspoon of Friar's balsam has been added. Alternatively paint the toes with neat Friar's balsam.

● *Tincture of myrrh* Paint this on to the toes or fingers.

● *Essence of horse chestnut* Diluted in a warm water footbath this will ease irritation and also stimulate circulation.

● *Elderflowers* Use elderflowers either in a decoction to rinse or bathe or in a hand cream. An elderflower compress will reduce pain.

● *Marigold flowers* An infusion of marigold flowers with 1 tablespoon of sea salt added to a bowl of warm water is very therapeutic.

Poultices and Ointments

The following remedies are based not only on the gentle warmth of the vegetable but also on the healing elements they contain. Potatoes, carrots, turnips and parsnips all contain vitamins C and B, phosphorus and potassium. Many of the remedies which incorporate root vegetables come from those areas in which such crops were grown and gathered. Planting and gathering root vegetables was a cold, dirty and back-breaking business which left the skin filthy and broken. Now farming methods may have improved but the old remedies are as effective today as they were a hundred years ago.

The cream for aches and pains to be found under **Rheumatism** is excellent for massaging painful chilblains provided they are not broken.

● *Potato poultice* Take 1 large, old potato baked in its jacket. Scrape out the pulp, mash well and apply to the toes and fingers as hot as is easily bearable. Leave until cool then wash off and pat dry. Rub in a suitable oil or cream. Do this nightly before bed and if possible wear gloves and bedsocks: not only do they protect painful hands and feet but they keep them warm which is particularly necessary for the elderly and very young whose circulation is often poor.
● *A beneficial potato paste for the hands* Mix 1 tablespoon each of almond oil and glycerine and 1 teaspoon of orange flower water to a paste with the mash of 2 baked potatoes. This will whiten hands damaged by heavy manual work or washing and gardening if spread on and left for an hour. It also soothes and heals chilblains, split fingers and swollen joints.

● *Figs and honey* Fresh roasted figs ground with honey and applied as a paste to chilblained fingers is a soothing and luxurious remedy. Poultices of strawberries were another extravagant favourite amongst the elite.
● *Oatmeal poultice* Warm porridge oats are amazingly effective and comforting if you can think how to keep the mixture on! Children will thoroughly enjoy sitting with their fingers in a bowl of warm goo however.
● *Groundsel, chickweed, comfrey* Any of these common green herbs made into a warm poultice will ease the pain of chilblains. Groundsel and chickweed grow prolifically where potatoes have been harvested and geese and chickens thrive on these two herbs. This example of practical smallholding also extended itself to healing because a vivid green ointment made by simmering a large quantity of groundsel in goose or chicken fat was considered to be the most healing unguent for chilblains and broken skin on hands and feet. In East Anglia where it was most commonly needed it was known as sinnon ointment.

Another Old-fashioned Ointment
225g(8oz) pure lard
75g(3oz) beeswax
600ml(1 pint) sweet almond oil
90ml(3 fl oz) oil of turpentine

Melt together the lard and beeswax. Warm the sweet almond oil and oil of turpentine together then beat into the lard mixture. Continue beating until the mixture is cool and emulsified. Pot, seal and keep refrigerated. Use on chilblains and chaps. This is a very old-fashioned recipe which does work but if you have reservations about using lard you can use white wax (paraffin wax) instead.

● *Marigold leaves* A warm poultice on a damaged digit will bring relief. So too will calendula oil or ointment.

Marigold Jelly
6 fresh marigold heads
1 large jar white petroleum jelly
(vaseline)

Clean and break up the flower heads. Melt the petroleum jelly in a bain-marie, add the marigolds and leave the mixture to simmer gently for several hours. Strain the mixture and pot. This is a very effective remedy for chilblains and cracked, sore skin on hands and feet. It also soothes hangnails and sunburn.

● *Elderflowers* The best possible hand cream for those suffering from chilblains can be made by simmering 225g(8oz) each of elderflowers and lard for half an hour then straining and potting the result. This is also an effective treatment for insect bites.

The Pains and Prerogatives of Womanhood

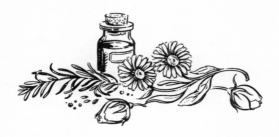

I am not an arrant feminist by any means but whilst I have been researching this book one thing has become abundantly clear and that is that as far as the old sages and practitioners of 'medicine' were concerned women were put on earth to suffer in the cause of producing a good home, a warm bed and many heirs for their menfolk, and what they may have had to suffer in the course of doing this was nothing more nor less than the cost of this privilege. This precept has unfortunately percolated down through the generations and many women still find themselves banging their heads against a wall of indifference erected by unscrupulous pharmaceutical companies and less than sympathetic practitioners. Against this argument one has

to say that no one would deny the tremendous progress made to ensure, for example, that more babies are born with a chance of survival.

Nevertheless when the chips are down on the more trivial yet totally debilitating aspects of womanhood the wise old women knew a thing or two about ensuring that their sisters were made more comfortable with the minimum of risk.

Period Pains

Some fortunate women suffer no more than three days of minor inconvenience whilst others endure a week of miserable cramps, headaches, sickness and heavy bleeding. There are a great many reasons for feeling rotten, all of which have been thoroughly discussed in every magazine and book on the subject. Water retention leads to a bloated feeling, weight gain and swollen ankles and puts pressure on the liver and kidneys. Stress, depression, sleeplessness and headaches not surprisingly follow in the wake of these miseries, especially if your face has sprouted its monthly crop of acne and the hair is lank and lifeless. Backache and cramp can also be caused by back problems so do not suffer needlessly but take the advice of an osteopath and ignore the concept popular amongst our male counterparts that woman is a menstruating biped with backache.

Bad temper is fairly understandable but this can flare into the unreasonable aggression associated with severe premenstrual tension. If you think that this is your problem find a sympathetic expert to advise you.

To bolster yourself against this monthly subversion from within take the following steps. Avoid coffee, tea, alcohol, stimulants, chocolate, junk food and unrefined carbohydrates. Eat a high-protein diet and lots of fresh fruit and vegetables, particularly spinach, dandelion leaves, carrots, apples and lady's mantle which will replace lost minerals and vitamins. Iron-rich liver is also recommended. Drink lots of water.

Take plenty of exercise – walking, swimming and yoga are the best.

Take vitamin B$_6$ or evening primrose in the eight to 10 days prior to a period but do not extend the course further. Take marigold tisane for one week before a period is due (see page 155). Magnesium, calcium and zinc may be taken as a supplement to relieve muscle tension whilst royal jelly, pollen and honey will further ease your tribulations. All of these sensible and gentle remedies are preferable to a dose of ergot of rye in water, opium and camphor or strong vinegar and horseradish sniffed up the nose to shake you out of your unseemly lethargy.

Effective Pain Killers

The following teas should all be made in the quantities of 1 teaspoon infused in 1 cup of boiling water for 10 minutes and taken three times a day unless stated otherwise.

- *Motherwort* The oldest and gentlest of female herbs, this will rid you of a headache. Take after meals.
- *Melilot* This is the sweet yellow or bee's clover. Take for headache and wring out in a compress for aching eyes.
- *Vervain* Sip this tea for headache and tension.
- *Dandelion* Take dandelion tea to alleviate water retention and a heavy bloated feeling.
- *Red raspberry leaf* Drink three times a day to relieve distention.
- *Cramp bark* Recommended for cramps and tension.
- *Fennel* This will ease pain, tension and digestive problems.
- *Camomile* Take for pain, stress and headache with a scanty period.
- *Pennyroyal* Another tea for a scanty period with pain.
- *Caraway* This tea relieves a cold bloated feeling and indigestion.
- *Angelica* Use to relieve pain, stress and digestive problems.
- *Yarrow* Take if you suffer from excessive bleeding, cramp and tension.
- *Strawberry leaf* This is another remedy for excessive bleeding.
- *Fresh fig leaves* An infusion of fresh fig leaves will improve the circulation.
- *Parsley and tarragon* Eat these herbs or make them into a tea.

• *Rose* Use the petals of the wild or white garden rose. One drop of essential oil in hot water is very soothing and tranquillizing.

• *Safflower or linseed* Steep 7g(¼oz) of the seeds in 600ml(1 pint) of boiling water, stand for five minutes then strain and drink 1 teacupful every five hours to reduce pain.

• *Peppermint, fennel and liquorice* Infuse peppermint leaves and fennel seeds in liquorice water and drink. Alternatively make a tea of the first two and eat liquorice wood or sweets. If constipation and water retention are the cause of pain it will help.

A Tea to Ease Period Pains
15g(½oz) each melilot and camomile flowers
15g(½oz) each mint and orange leaves
15g(½oz) each lime flowers and valerian root

Mix the ingredients together and add 1 teaspoon to 500ml(17 fl oz) of boiling water. Stand for five minutes then strain. Starting eight days before and for the duration of the period drink three cups over 24 hours. It can be taken hot or cold, with or without honey. This will ease cramps and pain and help to reduce stress.

A Strengthening Tonic for Women
3 tablespoons juniper berries
700ml(1¾ pints) water
1 teaspoon each camomile and comfrey tea
1 piece liquorice root

Soak the juniper berries in cold water for 15 minutes. Bring the water to the boil, add the drained berries to it and simmer until the liquid is reduced by one third. Discard the berries. Put the remaining ingredients into a warm china tea pot then reheat the juniper liquid to boiling point and pour it into the pot. Cover and leave to stand for five minutes. Take ½ cup four times a day.

A More Physical Approach

A forthright though not altogether practical suggestion comes from a very old herbal which advocates sitting over a bowl of steaming yarrow or tansy tea to relieve the pains and cramps of menstruation. A warm bath however, especially a warm sitz bath, will do much to ease the 'torsions and screws'. Add essential oils of orange blossom or orange, camomile, melissa or rose to the water. Also use them in a carrier oil to gently massage your aching tum, back and neck and the soles of your feet. Tell yourself that you love yourself, even if no one else does, and retire to bed with a hot-water bottle on your stomach, a pillow beneath your knees, a good book and the best but not very herbal remedy of gin and peppermint cordial in a splash of hot water. Port and brandy is another very therapeutic dram – but take no more than that! Great-grand-mothers may remember the alternatives of a hot compress and hot milk with grated nutmeg.

See also under **Cramps**, **Anxiety**, **Constipation**, **Headache**, **Problems of Digestion**, **Skin Disorders and Irritations**, and **A Healthy Head of Hair**.

THE MENOPAUSE

How we fight against it and how we dread it. Our mothers spoke of 'the change of life' in hushed whispers as though it were the plague itself come to visit us. Yet why should we dread it?

The physical problems associated with the menopause are usually no more or less than those endured during our normal periods though more erratic. The physical changes can be counteracted by more advanced thinking on diet, cosmetics and lifestyle. Think how much happier you will be when you no longer have 'the curse' or the fear of unwanted pregnancy and, unless you have a beady eye out for a toy boy, your husbands are ageing along with you. If you already have their love and respect you are not going to lose it overnight because you have one or two more wrinkles or the odd grey hair, and if bits do look in danger of dropping off or sagging beyond redemption that is probably your own fault for not having taken care in the past so you will have to work harder now.

What is unfair is that our own self-inflicted punishment and neurosis at this time can turn our loving families away from us because they just do not understand why a good and happy mother and partner has so suddenly changed. This can cause far greater unhappiness to everyone than is necessary. In this modern age women in their middle years are holding down high-powered jobs, carving new careers for themselves, finding creative hobbies and travelling extensively because all these options are open to them and they do not have to think about putting their families first. It is the time of their life. To many women, no matter how much they miss the mixed blessings of motherhood, this is a new-found and welcome freedom.

Nowadays our diets can be boosted with mineral and vitamin supplements to ensure that our faculties are kept intact and our bones strong. Looking and feeling good is not vanity: it is our right. Whilst we all have to work hard at it ourselves it is also worth examining hormone replacement therapy as an optional extra to boost good health and natural vitality once we have passed the so-called hurdle of the menopause.

To Help You Over the 'Hurdle'

- *Sage tonic* 'The desire of sage is to render man immortal.' Now whilst I cannot exactly guarantee the truth of this I can suggest that sage tea and the following tonic will make you feel much more chirpy. Take 100g(4oz) of fresh sage leaves and leave them to stand in a bottle of good white wine made by natural, not chemical, processes, for two weeks. Sweeten to taste with honey and leave for a further day. Press and strain through a cloth. Bottle and take 1 sherry glass before lunch and dinner.
- *Lemon balm* 'I tell 'ee boor I gave that old defoliated bird some of that there lemon stuff and blow me if 'er didn't grow new feathers and lay like no tomorrer.' What is good enough for the countryman is good enough for me. Melissa or lemon balm is reputed to ease the pains of the menopause, physically and mentally as well as increase fertility. The tea will soothe and the leaves under the pillow will bring tranquillity. A few drops of essential oil in the bath would not come amiss either.
- *Oil of cypress* Barberry and cypress tea is an old-fashioned remedy from France. The essential oil however, dropped into a warm bath or on to a hot compress to be held on the tum, is very soothing, and you might also like to add it to sunflower oil and massage with it. It will also reduce excess perspiration and foot odour.
- *Meadowsweet tea or hop tea* Both are soothing and reduce tension.
- *Mugwort tea* Mugwort is the plant

of the moon and of Artemisia, the patron saint of women. The tea drunk only in moderation will help you feel less hurt and weary. Carry a spray of the herb with you always to the same end.
• *Tansy tea or pennyroyal tea* These will stop the 'flushes'.
• *Marigold tea* Drink the tea regularly to ease menopausal disorders. Infuse 75g(3oz) of the flower heads in 1 litre(1¾ pints) of boiling water for 10 minutes. Drink 3 to 4 cups daily. Calendula tincture may also prove helpful.

Look under **Period Pains** for further advice.

PAINFUL CONDITIONS OF THE BREASTS

Whilst researching this book I have been led to the uneasy conclusion that most of the ancient physicians were men who regarded women purely in the role of child bearers and wet nurses. Midwives and wise women were far kinder to their suffering sisters, prescribing such soothing lotions and potions as belladonna fomentations, violet salve and herbal teas, whilst the best, or worst that their male counterparts could conjure up were baked turnip or goose dung mixed with celandine. Conditions which affect the breast however are not particularly amusing. Mastitis or 'hard breasts' is excruciatingly painful, causing pain in the area of arm and neck as well as inflaming and hardening the breast, and it inevitably creates anxiety in the mind that something worse may be indicated. Any lump or bump in the breast should always be a sign to take immediate professional advice.

Sore, cracked nipples are usually a result of breast feeding, either because of the baby dragging at the nipple or because the correct care is not being taken in washing and drying the breasts before and after feeding. It does cast a pall over what should be a satisfactory maternal experience.

Soothing Lotions and Potions

Mallows were believed to increase the supply and flow of milk as were borage, watercress, parsley, fennel, anise, hop, caraway, cumin, dill, carrots, lentils, milk thistle (recognized in the doctrine of signatures as a milk-bearing plant), love-in-a-mist and fenugreek which had the added benefit of giving the breasts an alluring roundness. Many of these herbs have the added benefit of counteracting post-natal depression. Vervain tea, 1 teaspoon infused in 1 cup of boiling water for 10 minutes, will also alleviate those dispirited feelings if taken three times a day. Half a teaspoon of sage infused in 1 cup of boiling water and drunk three times a day has the reverse effect of drying up the flow of milk.

To prevent sore and cracked nipples which can make feeding your baby an unhappy experience rub the nipples with a mixture of pure lemon juice and olive oil throughout your pregnancy and whilst you are nursing add a few drops of essential oil of geranium to a pot of cold cream and soothe the nipples with this. Calendula ointment may also help.

• *Marsh mallow and common mallow* Both of these are mentioned frequently in time-honoured herbal remedies and in the chauvinistic words of one Dr William Coles, a 17th century physician, 'for the Breasts and Paps of women – to procure a great flow of milk and to assuage the hardening thereof' take mallows boiled and buttered. Whether he meant as food or poultice I do not know. However a salve made from 50g(2oz) of the leaves and flowers of the common mallow simmered in 3 tablespoons of lard on white petroleum jelly (vaseline) is soothing and harmless.

Healing Massage Oil for the Breasts
4 tablespoons apricot oil
4 tablespoons wheatgerm oil

Shake together and use warm to massage painful breasts. If used warm it is even more soothing. Apricot oil smoothes wrinkles out and is used for this purpose in cosmetics.

Other Soothing Suggestions

- *Camphor* A few drops of oil of camphor in 2 tablespoons of olive oil may be used to massage 'hard breasts' but not when nursing.
- *Honey and olive oil or lanolin* Use honey and olive oil to anoint cracked nipples. Lanolin rubbed into the nipples also soothes and softens but do first make sure that you are not allergic to it.
- *Warm poultices* These are a standard and comforting remedy for mastitis hence the varied suggestions ranging from baked potatoes, turnips, fresh cooked – not baked – beans pounded with olive oil, hot plasters and warm fomentations to the unlikely and delightful thought of keeping one's breast in a 'sling'. A good, properly fitted, supporting bra will do however.

A Soothing Tea to Improve the Flow of Milk
1 teaspoon each dried aniseed, dill and marjoram
½ teaspoon dried fenugreek
600ml(1 pint) boiling water
honey

Infuse the herbs in the water for 10 minutes and sweeten with honey to taste if necessary. A poor flow of milk was always considered to be one of the causes of mastitis in nursing mothers.

PREGNANCY

Pregnancy and childbirth have to be the most natural things in the world but if you feel unwell do not try self-diagnosis or self-help but seek professional advice. It is not a good idea to take any potions, herbal or otherwise, when you are pregnant unless they have been specifically prescribed for you. The following remedies are merely external and will make you feel more comfortable. It is also essential that you eat the right foods when you are pregnant and most particularly that you avoid junk foods, alcohol and smoking.

It is a well known fact that pregnant women should look only on beautiful things and be at peace so that their child may be born contented.

Tea and a sweet plain biscuit before you sit up or move a foot out of bed in the morning will help prevent morning sickness.

Orange juice with honey or a few drops of orange flower water in warm water at night will help you sleep.

To prevent varicose veins do not stand still for long periods of time but do plenty of gentle walking. Do not wear restrictive clothing. Do put your legs up – a pillow under the feet in bed at night and legs up on a stool or pouffe when sitting. Swim if you can.

● *Herbal teas* The only, very mild, infusions that I would suggest are lime or camomile for insomnia and tension. They will also relieve morning sickness as will meadowsweet and peppermint. If you suffer from morning sickness consistently find out whether you are deficient in vitamin E or B but do nothing until advised by your practitioner.

● *Honey both for yourself and for your baby* It is believed that any baby brought up on honey from birth will avoid many of the problems associated with allergies and be strengthened against infection.

● *Massage oils* All through pregnancy and after the baby is born gently massage the stomach, breasts and thighs with olive or sunflower oil to ensure that stretch marks are kept to a minimum. Massage the legs upwards from the ankle to prevent varicose veins. Use the following therapeutic oil: 3 drops of essential oil of cypress and 2 drops each of lavender and lemon mixed into 1 eggcupful of sunflower oil. Massage the soles of the feet for utter relaxation. A special formula to keep breasts firm is to add 1 drop each of essential oils of rose and orange to an eggcup of apricot oil and use this to massage with. It will also promote peaceful thoughts.

Apricot Massage Cream (for use after the baby is born)
1 tablespoon each anhydrous lanolin and cocoa butter
2 tablespoons apricot oil
1 tablespoon orange flower water
½ teaspoon borax
a few drops of essential oil of orange flower

Melt the lanolin and cocoa butter together in a bowl in a bain-marie then stir in the warm apricot oil. Warm the orange flower water to the same temperature in a separate bowl and dissolve the borax in it. Beat the water into the oils and continue beating until the mixture is cool. Add the essential oil and spoon this fluffy, gloriously scented cream into a dry, clean pot. Seal tightly. Apricot oil has an excellent softening effect on wrinkles and slightly sagging skin so make use of it where weight loss is greatest after the baby is born.

VAGINAL THRUSH

There are two not dissimilar conditions which affect women: one is leucorrhoea (whites) and the other is the dreaded thrush which, it would seem, has only recently sprung into notoriety. Both of them have more or less the same symptoms – a vaginal discharge, fiery pain and fierce irritation. There is also pain in groin and abdomen caused by the glands swelling in sympathy. Some practitioners believe that the condition is contagious and therefore you would be wise to seek professional advice in the first instance. After that most of the answer is in self-help.

Stress, allergic reaction, excesses of junk food, alcohol, stimulant drinks and yeast can all cause what is basically an incorrect balance of flora in the gut, colon or vagina. In the case of thrush this flora is known as candida, a pretty name for a beastly nuisance. It is a fungal parasite which most of the time lies peaceably undisturbed in the colon and is kept in check by the immune system but it can, in the most simplistic terms, be stimulated into action by the use of antibiotics and the hormone pill. The many problems it may cause range from the physical to the psychological.

In the past herbalists prescribed herbal teas and douches as a method of controlling leucorrhoea and associated complaints but little modern research has been done to find an answer to thrush. There have been remedies but because they were non-profitable they have been dropped from professional use. Cystitis has often been thought to cause thrush but in effect it may be the antibiotics given to relieve this painful condition which actually do the damage, so if you are ever taking antibiotics for any reason at all also eat copious amounts of plain live yoghurt. Whilst our grandmothers, to protect us against these female complaints, would have advised us most strongly against eating fermenting jam or bread with mould on it, modern practitioners believe that tea, coffee, alcohol, chocolate, sugar, bread and mushrooms will also all exacerbate thrush.

Self-Help

Do not wear tight synthetic knickers and tights or figure-hugging jeans.

Whilst you have thrush do not attempt to enjoy the pleasures of sex. It will not be much fun anyhow.

When you go to the lavatory always wipe yourself from front to back to avoid spreading infection – how many women can remember their mothers instilling this precept into them from early childhood?

The best ways of easing the irritation and helping to clear the condition are to eat a pot of live yoghurt every morning and raw oats once a day and to take garlic perles or capsules daily.

Wash thoroughly every morning and night with a weak solution of hydrogen peroxide, dab gently dry on a tissue (throw it down the lavatory afterwards) and smear well with white petroleum jelly (vaseline). It wrecks your undies but prevents the discharge causing intense aggravation.

● *Nasturtium* An infusion made from nasturtium is a natural antibiotic and may serve well for washing with.

Before you rush off for professional advice on the cause or source of this unbelievable thing which has happened to you, do check first that you have not inadvertantly forgotten to remove a tampon!

● *Evening primrose oil* Take this to relieve stress rather than a vitamin B_6 tablet which may be yeast based.

● *Live yoghurt* As well as eating this daily it is suggested that a little can be inserted into the vagina on a tampon.

● *Honey* Take it alone or in apple cider vinegar every morning.

● *Blackberry leaf tea* This tea is to be taken for cystitis, piles and leucorrhea as well as for thrush.

● *Essential oils of juniper and lavender* Add either of these oils to the bath.

WATER RETENTION AND CELLULITE

These two are not the same things but when I was niggling about my somewhat dimpled thighs they were thus explained to me. When we are teenagers all these areas are filled up with puppy fat and over the following years they provide handy pockets for the excess water that the female body produces, eventually becoming more solid and hence the dimpling. It is no modern phenomenon but at one time mothers, matrons and middle-aged ladies did not disport themselves in bikinis in competition with the skinny, attenuated limbs of anorexic model girls. Therefore the answer is to attend to the water retention and keep the danger of the 'orange peel' dimples of cellulite to a minimum. Tiredness, stress, constipation and bad circulation can also cause water retention.

Diet

Do not eat too much salty or refined food or whole milk but have lots of fresh fruit, vegetables and high-protein foods and plenty of vitamin C.

● *Coffee and tea* Although they are diuretic they exacerbate the problem so reduce them to the minimum and drink a lot of water. It cleanses and purifies and will improve the body tone.
● *Exercise* Keep in trim and keep the circulation in top form.
● *Lemon* The rind boiled in water and left overnight is particularly good – a glass first thing in the morning works wonders. Home-made lemonade and lemon barley water are recommended too (see page 126).
● *Grapes and grape juice* A one-day fast on a grape diet will drain the water from you!

● *Kelp* Take kelp into your diet and use it in the bath. In conjunction with a bit of brisk brushing with a loofah it will perk up the circulation.
● *Dandelion tea* This is the best way to rid the body of excess water. Sage tea also helps. Eat both in a good green salad.
● *Lettuce and chervil tea* Use 25g(1oz) of lettuce leaf and 15g($\frac{1}{2}$oz) of chervil infused in 500ml(scant pint) of boiling water for 10 minutes and drink 3 cups a day as a prime remedy for water retention, cellulite, piles and varicose veins.
● *Onion soup* A warming onion soup brings good health – add sage for extra benefit and do not make it with milk.
● *Ivy* Cellulite can erupt into swollen rather inflamed patches which ache and become sore. If you have areas which pose such a problem here are two successful remedies which are as old as the hills. Chop 2 handfuls of common ivy leaves and mix with 4 handfuls of bran and enough warm water to form a paste. Apply as a poultice (it is also used on horses with oedema). Boil 150g(5oz) of chopped ivy leaves in 1 litre(1$\frac{3}{4}$ pints) of water for 10 minutes and apply on a compress.

LIST OF SUPPLIERS

This is by no means a comprehensive list of suppliers of the raw materials which are used in this book but includes those that I have found to be consistently reliable and helpful.

Local pharmacies Most local chemists stock old-fashioned syrups and mixtures. They also keep small quantities of rose water, whitch hazel, tincture of arnica and so on. I hope that you may find them as helpful as I have found my own local pharmacists, Michael and Ann Farrell and Mr. Spencer, to have have been.

Ready-made herbal preparations:
Sunshine Health Supplies,
25 Church Street,
Stroud,
Gloucestershire GL5 1JL
Tel. 01453 751395
Postal service and personal shoppers

Herbs, oils, waxes, health foods and drinks:
G. Baldwin & Co. Medical Herbalists,
171/173 Walworth Road,
London SE17 1RW
Tel. 0171–703 5550
Postal service and personal shoppers

Waxes, oils, powders, creams and herbs:
John Bell and Croyden,
52/54 Wigmore Street,
London W1
Tel. 0171–935 5555
Postal service and personal shoppers

Herbs and herbal products:
Culpepers – many branches for personal shoppers.
Postal service:
Culpeper Ltd.,
Hadstock Road,
Linton,
Cambridge CB1 6NJ
Tel. 01223 891196

Neal's Yard Apothecary,
15 Neal's Yard,
Covent Garden, London WC2
Tel. 0171-379 7222
and
Corn Market Street, Oxford

Seeds for growing your own herbs:
Chiltern Seeds,
Bortree Stile,
Ulverston,
Cumbria LA12 7PB
Tel. 01229 581137

Organically grown produce:
Food From Britain,
123 Buckingham Palace Road,
London SW1W 9FA
Food From Britain produce a book, *Food Focus*, and issue information on all sources of organically produced foodstuffs available throughout the British Isles.

Advice on obtaining and growing herbs:
The Herb Society,
Deddington Hill Farm,
Warmington,
Banbury OX17 1XB

Index of Ailments

INDEX OF REMEDIES